Further praise for

Happiness in a Storm

"Dr. Harpham mixes practical advice with a deep concern for each and every Healthy Survivor. She brings all her firsthand experience as doctor, patient, and *very* Healthy Survivor to bear on the most essential of human values—the pursuit of happiness. This book is a great asset to all—patient, caregiver, and physician interested in navigating the course to Healthy Survivorship."
—Leonard Zwelling, MD, MBA, vice president of research administration, MD Anderson Cancer Center

"This book pulses with the fervent heart and knowledge that its author brings as both patient and physician. The joy that Wendy Harpham has found in learning to live with cancer, whatever the outcome, is illuminated by a cogent argument for hope that is the most compelling I have ever encountered."—Joanna Bull, MA, founder, Gilda's Club Worldwide

"Wendy Harpham has written a wonderful book. Her understanding of the impact of serious illness on people—how it changes lives, relationships, perspective on the world, thinking and feeling, and just about everything else—is nothing less than extraordinary. The advice she gives about what patients should do about their care and themselves is practical, solid, and, above all, useful. On top of that, she is a wise, knowledgeable, upbeat, and caring woman, and that shines through on every page. Her book is must reading for people and families threatened by serious disease. It is just as valuable for physicians, nurses, and other caregivers who will find it very helpful and more than worth their time."—Eric J. Cassell, MD, MACP, clinical professor of public health, Weill Medical College of Cornell University

"Wendy Schlessel Harpham's important new book, *Happiness in a Storm*, is frank, realistic, scientific, and up-to-date, but most important it will be helpful—even to people who say they have lost hope for a fulfilling life after a serious illness. 'Healthy survivorship is an art,' Dr. Harpham writes, 'and like all art you won't find an absolute 'right' or 'wrong' way to do it.' With *Happiness in a Storm*, Wendy Schlessel Harpham has turned the 'How-To' book into an art form."—Natalie Robins, author of *A Cancer Journal*

"*Happiness in a Storm* is a warm, knowledgeable, and personal exploration of living with illness. Dr. Harpham presents wise and clear advice about riding the emotional roller coaster that is life with illness. She teaches how to hope for the best but prepare for the worst, respect your emotions and learn from them. Her book is heartwarming because she shows how she faces sadness and uncertainty while celebrating her son's home runs and her husband's love for her. Dr. Harpham makes the phrase 'tears of joy' understandable."
—David Spiegel, MD, Willson Professor and medical director, Center for Integrative Medicine, Stanford University, and author of *Living Beyond Limits*

"As I read Wendy Harpham's *Happiness in a Storm*, I felt as though she were walking beside me, encouraging, appreciating, and informing me on how to undertake the journey through cancer-land with all my courage and optimism in hand. She covers all aspects of the experience from the practical and medical through the emotional and spiritual. Everyone facing illness would do well to read this book."—Susan P. Halpern, MSW, author of *The Etiquette of Illness: What to Say When You Can't Find the Words*

"*Happiness in a Storm* gives us just what we need to face illness with knowledge, action, and hope. Rarely do we get perspective from a physician who is not only a medical expert but also a survivor with a compassionate, resilient soul. Thanks to Wendy Harpham, we now have a book filled with practical tips and medical guidance with inspiration woven throughout. It's one of those books we will carry with us everywhere. Thanks to Wendy for guiding us to face illness and remember life's joys available to each of us in any storm."—Jackie Waldman, author of *The Courage to Give* series

"Dr. Wendy Harpham's writings tell it all as to the kind of person/doctor she is. Hope is sometimes all we have to keep us going. Many thanks to Wendy."
—Kathleen Williams, CMA, CST, survivor of ruptured brain aneurysm

"A jewel of a book and a gift to all who are confronting a serious illness. Wendy Schlessel Harpham draws on her personal experience as a physician and cancer survivor to offer empowering words of wisdom, inspiration, and hope to others who are 'living through' cancer. Dr. Harpham's resilience and generosity of spirit are truly awe-inspiring."—JoAnn E. Manson, MD, DrPH, chief, Division of Preventive Medicine, Brigham and Women's Hospital; professor of medicine, Harvard Medical School

happiness in a storm

Also by Wendy Schlessel Harpham, MD

Diagnosis: Cancer:
Your Guide to the First Months of Healthy Survivorship

After Cancer:
A Guide to Your New Life

When a Parent Has Cancer:
A Guide to Caring for Your Children,
with the illustrated children's book,
Becky and the Worry Cup

The Hope Tree: Kids Talk about Breast Cancer
co-authored with Laura Numeroff

happiness in a storm

*Facing Illness
and Embracing Life
as a Healthy Survivor*

Wendy Schlessel Harpham, MD

W. W. Norton & Company
New York · London

Our knowledge about illness and healing is constantly changing. This book is not intended as a substitute for competent medical care. It serves to supplement the information provided by your doctors and nurses.

While the incidents in this book are true, I have changed particulars or people's names, or occasionally created composites to protect privacy.

For information about permission to reproduce selections from this book, write to
Permissions, W. W. Norton & Company, Inc., 500 Fifth Avenue, New York, NY 10110

Manufacturing by RR Donnelley, Harrisonburg, VA
Book design by Chris Welch Design
Production manager: Andrew Marasia

Library of Congress Cataloging-in-Publication Data

Harpham, Wendy Schlessel.
Happiness in a storm : facing illness and embracing life as a healthy survivor /
Wendy Schlessel Harpham.— 1st ed.
p. cm.
Includes index.
ISBN 0-393-06080-2 (hardcover)
1. Sick—Attitudes. 2. Sick—Psychology. 3. Chronically ill—Attitudes.
4. Chronic diseases—Psychological aspects. 5. Happiness. I. Title.
R726.5.H37 2005
155.9'16—dc22

2005011983

W. W. Norton & Company, Inc., 500 Fifth Avenue, New York, N.Y. 10110
www.wwnorton.com

W. W. Norton & Company Ltd., Castle House, 75/76 Wells Street, London W1T 3QT

1 2 3 4 5 6 7 8 9 0

*To the researchers and clinicians who are dedicated
to helping patients become Healthy Survivors.*

*To the researchers and clinicians
who saved my life and cared for me.*

The sea, like life itself, is a stern taskmaker. The best way to get along with either is to learn all you can, then do your best and don't worry, especially about things over which you have no control.

—Admiral Chester William Nimitz, quoting his grandfather in E. B. Potter's Nimitz

Contents

Acknowledgments

One of my greatest joys as a writer is receiving candid comments on my manuscripts. Without this critical feedback from my select group of "readers," how could I know if my meaning is clear, tone is comforting, or message is helpful to others?

My most dedicated and valuable reader is my husband. Thank you, Ted, for seven and a half years of listening to me work my way through the challenges of presenting medical information and my approach to survivorship. Thank you for reading innumerable drafts when the very last thing you wanted to think about was illness and healing. Most of all, thank you for twenty-five years (and counting) of "happily ever after," loving me the way you do, in sickness and in health.

Thank you James F. Strauss, MD, my oncologist, and Leonard Zwelling, MD, MBA, for reviewing and discussing chapters 2 and 6. Since closing my practice, I treasure any opportunity to talk about (and argue about) medical matters and their presentation to patients.

Thank you Brenda S. Casey, RN, my chemo nurse, and Adele M. O'Reilly, my dear friend, for reading the entire manuscript and for your enduring encouragement throughout the writing of this book.

Thanks to the many colleagues and friends who have given me the gift of reading my work-in-progress. Whether you read just a few pages of an early draft or one or two chapters of a later one, your response helped me move forward. With sincere apologies if I accidentally left out anyone, I thank Debra Sue Bruck, Clare Buie Chaney, PhD, Eileen Cole, M. Scott Daniel, MD, Barbara Ewing, Jean M. Harpham, Wendy Hobbie, CRNP, MSN, Barbara Hoffman, JD, Mary Jacobs, Robert Jones, Fannie Newman, Beth Lasher, Natalie Robins, Jane Ramberg, Joni Rodgers, Donna Ryan, Gabriel A. Shapiro, MD, Elizabeth Stein, Marvin J. Stone, MD, Nancy Taylor, Ruth Trimmer, Estelle Weissburg, Kathy Williams, and Sharon Witherspoon. To Joanna Bull, MA, MFCC, and Greta Greer, LCSW, CCM, thanks for reviewing the last appendix.

I'll always be grateful for the talented people at W. W. Norton, especially my editor, Amy Cherry, whose patience, attention to detail, and responsiveness can't be beat. Thank you, Amy, for nurturing my voice. And thank you, Faith Hamlin, for representing me, believing in this book, and taking care of the business end so I could focus on writing.

Rebecca Anne, Jessica Martha, and William Samuel have been watching me write this book for much of their lives. Thanks, kids, for cheering me on and having faith in me, even when you suspected that cows could fly before I finished this project. Thank you, thank you, thank you for bringing so much happiness into my life.

Prologue

It was the bottom of the last inning. The Blue Jays were behind by two runs. Not the Toronto Blue Jays baseball team but a group of second-grade boys from Dallas, some of whom hadn't yet grasped the concept of waiting for a good pitch. Nestled on the bleachers between my seriously sports-minded ten- and twelve-year-old daughters, I hugged one arm tight around Jessica and the other around Rebecca as my son watched me watch him stride from the dugout to home plate. "William can be the winning run!" I gasped, squeezing my girls even tighter.

"Dr. Harpham, I'm amazed."

A woman's voice from just behind my ear startled me, and I twisted around to see a woman whom I barely knew. She hesitated and, with a look of puzzlement, stumbled, "How can you be happy when you . . . ?"

Word spread quickly whenever I was back in treatment for the lymphoma that had been plaguing me since soon after my thirty-sixth birthday seven years earlier. Rarely were parents of my children's classmates and teammates unaware of my illness. Praise from anyone about how I was handling it usually made me squirm. Her comment was different from the others, arousing in me a spine-tingling awareness that, *yes: I am happy*.

My smile provided a graceful exit, allowing me to turn my back for full concentration on the baseball game. But my mind was distracted by memories of sitting on similar bleachers two years earlier, wearing a pasted-on smile in hopes of hiding what I was *really* thinking and feeling, namely, that I'd rather be almost anywhere else than in a place where people were supposed to be enjoying themselves. The mental images that followed formed a collage of bittersweet moments: dressing Rebecca for her ballet recital which I had to miss because of low blood counts, chatting with guests at my first book signing the evening before beginning radiation for my first recurrence, and giving my husband, Ted, humorous greeting cards and T-shirts in hopes of rescuing his forty-second birthday from the upheaval of my just-completed investigational treatment for a second cancer recurrence. These were special times that I had tried in earnest to enjoy but couldn't.

"Go, Will!"

My girls' cheers brought me back to the game. The umpire fed the ball into the pitching machine that hurled it toward the plate. In one smooth motion William swung, missed, and glanced up at me, looking for whatever it is that mothers supply little boys in batter's boxes.

"That's okay, Will. You can do it this time. Keep your eye on the ball!" I yelled encouragingly.

William wiggled the tip of his bat as the second pitch approached the plate. Again he swung, missed, and then looked to me as the ump signaled strike two.

"Hang in there, William. You only need to hit one," I screamed, giving him the thumbs-up sign.

I knew what was different. I knew why I was able to be in the middle of cancer treatments and feel happy, a combination that had seemed impossible when I was first diagnosed. I also knew that the key to my happiness didn't rest in some simple word or phrase but in how I lived my life after my illness. The roots of my approach to life as a patient sprouted long before a single defective lymphocyte in my body became cancerous and surreptitiously divided in two. Since my first days in medical school in 1976, I'd labored to understand life after diagnosis and treatment. In training and in my medical practice, I'd studied with fascination how heart disease, stroke, diabetes, spinal injuries, and countless other ailments altered not only patients' biology but also their lives. Occasionally while driving home I'd try to imagine what it must feel like to have one of the medical problems I'd seen that day, hoping for further insights into how to be a better doctor. My curiosity was peaked every time I saw patients with nearly identical diseases who received the same treatments yet achieved different medical outcomes. Clearly, the likelihood of a person's recovery depended on more than just choosing the right medicines. What made the difference? And what was the common thread linking my patients in difficult situations who exuded peacefulness or joy?

Fourteen years later, in 1990, cancer yanked me across the great divide from physician to patient. Specific memories of some patients' disasters and other patients' seemingly miraculous recoveries jumbled with the terrifying realization that I was seriously sick and had three young children to raise. The result was a mix of fear and inspiration. With Mamabear determination, I made myself a promise: *I will do whatever I have to do as a patient to increase my chance of surviving.*

That I was worried about surviving at all, let alone not living to a ripe old age, upset everything I'd accepted as normal. Having inherited my body type, high energy, and intensity from my mother (a seemingly invulnerable woman from a line of long-lived relatives), I'd assumed that I would outlive my husband, Ted. This expectation formed the fabric of my "normal" for as long as I could remember. Now this assumption had lost its relevance. With a crash, the cancer diagnosis interrupted my present and destroyed my confidence in my future. Out of yesterday's rubble, I had to find or create a new normal for today and a renewed faith in tomorrow.

Much as I yearned for reassurance that I would survive, my main goal was not long life. Trained to do battle against disease and death, in my medical practice I'd learned that a triumphant life is measured by *how* one lives, not how long. Caring for thousands of patients, I saw people find fulfillment and joy while others in similar circumstances lived in bitterness or despair. I had always wanted to believe that if illness or injury ever struck me, I'd be like those who could find happiness. Deep down, I feared that I wouldn't. During the dizzying days following my cancer diagnosis, I made a second promise to myself: *I will learn how to live my life most fully despite illness and maybe even because of it.* These two vows provided steadfast guidance and strength in what, for me, was to become an unwilling marriage with illness.

Once my cancer treatments began, keeping my pledge to do whatever I had to do was anything but romantic. Despite the advantage of my medical background, being an effective patient was complicated and draining, demanding much more than just knowing the right things to do. I had to learn how to have hope. And I had to learn how to act on my knowledge and hope. Even harder was discovering how to feel joy or a sense of fulfillment under the circumstances. Motivated by my pain, grief, and fear, I read and talked and listened and prayed in hopes of finding wisdom or mantras that could help me.

As I found ways to ease my own physical and emotional discomforts (or just to understand them better), I began to record information and advice that might help someone else. Witnessing other patients' confusion, struggles, sense of helplessness, and misplaced confidence in what I knew to be myth or misinformation ignited my sense of professional obligation. By stripping me of my white coat and stethoscope, cancer bared a new calling: writing for patients from the vantage of physician-survivor. I've been writing ever since.

My earlier books were all written while I was going through a series of remissions and recurrences that were treated with various courses of chemotherapy, radiation, immunotherapy, and antibody therapy in clinical trials. Illness for me was a lingering storm that descended with little warning, and that waxed and waned for years. My writing from those years reflects the chronic strain of treatment courses and protracted recoveries punctuated by times of high stress surrounding medical setbacks and routine checkups, when my hopes for cure and long life were tested with each delivery of bad news.

In searching for happiness while dealing with cancer, I gradually developed an approach to survivorship that helped me—and continues to help me—get good medical treatment and live as full a life as possible. This approach helped me face unpleasant statistics, so that I was able to make wise decisions and then nourish genuine hope that I'd land on the good side of the odds. It has helped me grieve losses so that I've been able to savor what remains and appreciate the many silver linings. It has encouraged me to accept my limits and then stretch them by pursuing the countless opportunities within my realistic choices. With many of my fears tamed, the knowledge of what might have been lost, and what might yet be, makes me feel today in a wonderfully intense way. My senses are freed to appreciate the coziness and sweet smell of a soft rain and the promise of rainbows. That summer at my son's Little League game, it was because of my practiced approach to survivorship that I could feel joy while dealing with the discomforts and uncertainty of cancer treatment.

In the late spring of 1997, I wrote an outline for this book that addresses the "why" behind the advice and mantras of my earlier books. The timing seemed perfect: The fact that my cancer was in remission would infuse my writing with the emotional high of renewal, yet provide a measure of objectivity not possible when I'm sick. In the months it would take to write a first draft, I could continue taking the steps necessary to speed my recovery at home so that I could return to work and maybe even practice medicine in some form.

To my surprise and disappointment, soon after completing the outline, my routine scans showed recurrent lymphoma. As always, I knew what I had to do to get a thorough and timely evaluation. Unlike after my first diagnosis, I also knew how to get things organized at home and what to say to my children. By now, I recognized the kaleidoscope of feelings that accompanied adjusting to the blinding news, and I took comfort in the knowledge that my emotions would smooth out with time. Even so, it was still an awful time until I slipped into my new routine that included treatments, checkups, Little League games, writing, longer naps, and support-group meetings.

At home after one of my treatments that summer, a friend of mine called me from the office of our mutual oncologist.

"Wendy," she choked, "It's . . . not . . . good."

Her Hodgkin's disease was back, even though she had passed the two-year mark after which patients in her particular situation usually breathe a little easier because their risk of recurrence drops. Her news shook me. Sad and mad, I offered love, prayers, and practical advice. Then I offered hope, telling her the story of William at bat.

With his team behind by two runs, and two teammates on base, William stood waiting after his first two strikes. The pitch came in. Once again William swung, only this time his bat connected. I really don't recall if it was a great hit or one of those that dribble past the outfielders. All I remember is standing in the bleachers with that wonderful lost-in-the-moment feeling, cheering with everyone as William rounded the bases with his arms stretched to the sky and a grin on his face. The Blue Jays won the game!

"In other words," I encouraged my frightened friend over the phone by quoting Yogi Berra, "It ain't over 'til it's over."

With months of treatment ahead of me, I wanted to use the time positively and not just wish it away. What better opportunity than to write about Healthy Survivorship? Writing would help me find and nourish the feeling I had at William's baseball game and allow me to share the feeling with others, such as my friend with Hodgkin's lymphoma facing another long course of chemotherapy and the healthy woman in the bleachers who simply couldn't understand my joy despite my illness. What I'd lost in objectivity when my cancer recurred I'd gained in immediacy. Feeling unwell, I was acutely aware of the uncertainty of my future. Clouds of possible pain, loss, and death darkened my horizon. Winds of fear and grief were blowing around me. Yet, even so, I felt far more confident in facing my future than during my first remission when I had talked of putting my illness completely behind me. This time around, as the first raindrops of treatment fell, I knew how to find happiness in a storm.

happiness in a storm

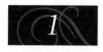

The Promise of Healthy Survivorship

I was driving alone to my oncologist's office in 1994 to have him check a lump I'd discovered while showering the previous evening. Pushing the buttons on my radio console in search of calming music, I heard an advertisement for a weekend getaway at a local hotel: "Do you want to escape the humdrum routine and add a little excitement to your life?" Responding aloud to the commercial voice, I yelled, "No! Don't you understand? 'Humdrum' sounds heavenly!" Let there be no doubts: I was committed to gaining every chance for recovery and willing to accept whatever blood tests, scans, procedures, and treatments were necessary. Yet, as my foot pushed down on the gas pedal, my heart longed for a normal life.

A diagnosis of serious illness disrupts your normal life. In one defining moment, you lose your sense of control of your world. The realization of potential losses sucks the air right out of you. You may fear losing a body part or function, your physical comfort, your livelihood, an important relationship, or your dreams for the future. Looming large, or lurking in the background, is the crucial question "Will I survive?" After the shock fades and raw fear no longer colors your vision, other questions arise: "When will my life feel normal again?" "How can I find happiness, now?"

As both a physician and long-term cancer survivor, I've seen patients for whom a diagnosis of serious disease marks a time after which everything seems to be a crisis, and joy has become foreign and unreachable. I've also seen ordinary people integrate unwanted challenges and losses into their lives. They embrace a "new normal," different from their old one, yet genuinely hopeful and, for the most part, happy. For some, the lessons learned through surviving illness make their new normal, in certain ways, even better than the way their lives were before.

Chances are you are reading this book because you or someone you love has a serious or chronic illness. The diagnosis may be new and stunning, or long-standing and as familiar as an old shoe. You may expect to be cured, or you may need a miracle to get better. Treatment may be an imminent trial, an ongoing effort, or a distant memory. Whatever the case, you want to find happiness in your life.

The quest for happiness is nothing new. The world's religions have been instructing generations how to cope with suffering and mortality. Philosophers have been advising how to find happiness in the face of difficulty and uncertainty. Much of the wisdom expressed in these teachings transcends time. The two-thousand-year-old dictum

While there's life, there's hope.

of the Roman philosopher Cicero "While there's life, there's hope" has comforted and inspired me through terrible times. Some patients have coped well by following the ancient tradition of remaining stoic rather than going along with today's popular approach of "letting it all out."

The problem is that the wisdom literature and great religions didn't address the complexities of being a patient in the twenty-first century. Philosophers and spiritual leaders couldn't imagine the unique stresses associated with participating in clinical trials, or the specific challenges of finding happiness during and after radiation, chemotherapy, organ transplants, placement of artificial body parts, or other high-tech treatments. Today's survivors find themselves trying to integrate these ancient teachings with their personal medical circumstances. While many succeed, too many others are left floundering: How much do I need to know? What choices do I have? How much of my life is under my control? How can I be happy under these circumstances?

From the time of my diagnosis on, I've believed that my own happiness as a cancer survivor has been tied to being a "Healthy Survivor," namely someone who is (1) getting good medical care while (2) living as fully as possible. Why? Good medical care helps me maximize my chances for recovery and keeps me as pain-free and functional as possible. By helping me feel calmer, more hopeful, and physically comfortable, good medical care puts me in a better position to enjoy life. And, although I believe that good medical care demands that I put in the time and energy required to be an effective patient, I also need to be able to forget about my illness at times. I can't be truly happy if cancer is always the central focus of my days. As a Healthy Survivor, I've worked hard to find a healthy balance—knowing when to pay attention to my illness and knowing when I can let it fade into the background.

In these pages, I share with you my approach to Healthy Survivorship, an outlook and a way of dealing with illness that is based on three steps: (1) obtaining sound knowledge, (2) finding and nourishing hope, and (3) acting effectively. This three-step approach has been guiding me through and beyond my disease for many years now. In every part of my life, this knowledge-hope-action approach has helped me increase my chances of a good outcome and, at the same time, live as fully as possible.

This book is for those of you who are trying to make your life the best it can be or, at least, better than it is now. In the setting of illness, sometimes the very best is not so great. In fact, as much as we'd all like to believe otherwise, your overall best may be worse than a low from before. Yet, even in terrible circumstances, you can experience great happiness *despite* your problems and losses, and sometimes even *because* of them. No matter what your situation is, you can get good care and live as fully as possible. In other words, you can become a Healthy Survivor.

Healthy Survivorship is an art. Like all art, you won't find an absolute "right" or "wrong" way to do it. Many factors unique to you—your needs, desires, strengths, weaknesses, goals, values, and circumstances— will determine what constitutes good medical care and what it means for you to live fully. Thankfully, you don't have to start from scratch. The experiences and insights of veteran survivors of serious illness can be useful when you are struggling. Hearing their stories can enlighten you, lift your spirits, and energize you. The trouble with relying solely on others' inspiration is that, after a few days or weeks, you'll be back where you were unless something fundamental has changed about your approach to dealing with your own situation.

Happiness in a Storm is not a story about me but a description and an explanation of my approach to life after my cancer diagnosis. I've written this as if you've invited me into your living room and asked me to share my thoughts about illness and healing, life and miracles in order to help you think about your own health, hopes, and happiness. I explain the knowledge-hope-action method that has helped me land on the good side of bad statistics and has guided me as I've gratefully grown older. Although my experience has been with cancer, all but a few specific points about cancer treatments apply equally well to dealing with any health crisis or challenge.

The first five chapters discuss what it means to heal after being diagnosed with serious illness or suffering an injury. I explain how knowledge about your illness helps you and offer a framework for organizing the confusing array of treatments. Throughout, I am encouraging you to take advantage of what science has to offer, helping you stack the odds in your favor and set the stage for the miracle of healing. The next four chapters are a more specific guide to optimizing your treatments and dealing with the emotional challenges of illness. But when it comes right down to it, what good is surviving if you are never happy? The last chapter is based on my belief that getting good care does more than increase your chances of an optimal medical outcome: It frees you to pursue happiness. The vulnerability, uncertainty, pain, and loss accompanying illness provide opportunities to know both the fragility and hopes of life and with this knowledge to live most fully. I encourage you to find and create happiness in your own life *despite* your medical problems, and to tap into the special happiness that can occur *because* of your illness. Although serious illness is bad, survivorship can lead you to meaningful and joyful times amid the hardships.

Use this book in whatever way meets your needs. You can read the chapters in order, or you can flip back and forth to specific chapters or subsections that address your current concerns. The italicized questions can help you think about each topic in terms of your own life. The knowledge-hope-action approach to Healthy Survivorship can help you appreciate the power you have to positively affect the course of your illness and move forward. My three-pronged approach is intended only as a springboard as you write your own story, developing and refining your own personal approach to Healthy Survivorship. I can't guarantee that you'll be cured of your disease, but I can promise this: Obtaining the right amount of knowledge, nourishing hope, and acting effectively can help you to get good care and live fully. At best, it will bring you comfort, hope, peace, and joy in good health.

Years ago, a radio announcer tried to tempt me with a weekend respite from the stresses and routines of normal life, as if the break would bring happiness. As a survivor, the last thing I want is to escape my life. I want to embrace it, every bit of it.

From Physician to Writer

After years of caring for patients in my solo practice of internal medicine, I was diagnosed with an indolent non-Hodgkin's lymphoma, a slow-growing cancer of the lymphatic system with no known cure. As was typical for patients with this disease who are treated aggressively, I had a good response to the initial course of chemotherapy, but my cancer recurred again and again over the subsequent eight years. Those years of my survivorship were times of terror, calm, desolation, almost mystical connection to others, confusion, clarity, sadness, and joy. Yet each round of diagnosis-treatment-recovery was unique because life around me changed from cycle to cycle, and so did I.

When I was first hospitalized in 1990 with excruciating leg pain and found to have cancer, my children were not quite two, four, and six years old. Rebecca, my oldest, remembers vaguely our precancer family life and vividly the turmoil surrounding my original diagnosis and the intensive treatments that followed. Jessica, my middle child, and William, my baby, have few memories of that terrible first year. For them, I've always had blue eyes, brown hair, and cancer. Able to discuss my disease in rather sophisticated terms long before they really understood what cancer was or why it was bad, each of my children found a place in their worldview for cancer in general and my lymphoma in particular. In doing so, their youthful honesty and optimism helped shape my outlook. Jessica gave me new insight into my medical situation when I overheard her say, "Sometimes she's in treatment, and sometimes she's on a 'mission,'" her term for remission. When a colleague was diagnosed with a similar lymphoma, Rebecca's immediate response was "You two can be survivors together!" a reaction in sharp contrast to that of every adult who learned the news.

Ted, my husband, is a philosophy-loving professor of political science. A voracious and passionate reader, after my diagnosis he found himself wandering in unfamiliar aisles of bookstores and libraries—the health and the religion sections. My illness gave new spin to the age-old questions he'd tackled professionally in the classroom: Why do bad things happen? What is the proper way to respond to adversity? What and where is God in all this? How much do we control what happens in our lives? What role do we play in our own happiness?

Ted's experience has been much different than mine. He stands on the shore of illness, firmly grasping my hand, watching the tide of disease try to pull me under and away from him. I've feared dying; he's pondered living on without me. Ted and I, whether brainstorming together or each lost in our private thoughts, keep wrestling with philosophies while negotiating the squalls of my illness. Each medical challenge has tested and reshaped our philosophies, exposing weaknesses and reinforcing strengths. All this time, we've never expected an ultimate resolution. We've hoped only to find practical and philosophical answers that can help us today.

Medical problems form the outline of my story, documented in physicians' charts and on X-ray films. Lymphoma, intensive treatments, infections, leg pain, and digestive problems characterized the first couple of years. Cancer recurrences, unbridled fear, sleep disturbances, and investigational treatments received far from home marked the next couple of years. Further recurrences, less toxic treatments, and persistent fatigue have characterized the last few years. My story is textured with the fallout of living with chronic disease: leaving a busy medical practice and becoming an at-home mom, adjusting to in-my-face awareness of my mortality and the fragility of life. Pain and uncertainty fractured my world. Philosophy, spirituality, and love glued the pieces back together.

For me, the biggest surprise of my survivorship is not that Ted and I have grown closer, that my children have grown stronger, or that my spiritual faith has grown deeper, but that I have turned to writing books.

> Philosophy, spirituality, and love are the glue that holds your life together in hard times.

Clinical medicine was my calling, one felt since I was a teenager. When cancer first forced me to take a ten-month medical leave from my solo medical practice, writing distracted me from the discomforts of treatment. My intention was to write a pamphlet for patients that summarized the information and advice I could offer as a physician-survivor. My nuts-and-bolts brochure grew into a published book, *Diagnosis: Cancer.*

After my chemotherapy was completed, and as soon as I was able, I put writing aside and returned to my "real" work: clinical medicine. Only eight months later, I was diagnosed with my first recurrence. Forced back into the cancer arena and unable to satisfy the inflexible demands of private practice, I closed my office for good. Looking for relief from my grief and sense of dislocation, I turned to the diversion that had grounded me before: writing for patients. A second remission of the lymphoma led to a job stint in another doctor's office, but my tenure was cut short by ill health and the need for more cancer treatments. I've yet to recover the physical stamina needed for clinical medicine. In the meantime, writing has become a different but equal passion and a way to reach more people than I ever could in my own office.

During the first five years of my cancer treatments, writing was therapeutic for me because working on patient-centered books and articles enabled me to feel like a doctor no matter what was happening medically. Back then, the challenge lay in finding clear and engaging ways to share with readers what was old hat to me: medical facts and practical advice. The past seven years of writing *Happiness in a Storm* have been different. In trying to explain and share examples of my personal approach to

Healthy Survivorship, I've wrestled with questions such as "What is my role in my own healing?" "How can I learn to feel brave in situations that frighten me?" "How do I narrow the gap between knowing what to do and actually doing it?" "How can I embrace today with all its limits while nourishing hope for a better tomorrow?" The search for clear answers that I could share in this book has led me to discover new meaning behind the tested philosophies, relationships, and faith of my survivorship. In doing so, writing *Happiness in a Storm* has helped me heal and encouraged me to pursue happiness. I now rarely think about what I've lost because I'm too busy focusing on what I've gained. Embracing the life I have today, I look forward to growing old and gray.

The Power of Healthy Survivorship

From the time of discovery and for the balance of life, an individual diagnosed with cancer is a survivor.—*Charter, National Coalition for Cancer Survivorship (1985)*

The introduction of the term *Survivor* was instrumental in helping transform cancer patients from silent victims of their disease to vocal participants in their care. With the power of words, "Survivor" helped lift the shroud of secrecy surrounding "the big C" and has helped patients and their loved ones focus on life not death, hope not despair, and power not victimization. All patients, not just cancer patients, have become less ashamed—even proud—of their survivorship.

You are a survivor the moment you are diagnosed. Knowing that you are a survivor gives you a hopeful starting stance for talking about your illness while feeling disoriented by the news and all the sudden changes prompted by the discovery of disease.

You are a survivor while undergoing evaluation. Knowing that you are a survivor gives you a hopeful platform for talking about your illness while adjusting to the diagnosis, undergoing evaluation, facing the statistics and uncertainty surrounding your treatment options, and deciding on a course of treatment.

You are a survivor while undergoing treatment. Knowing that you are a survivor gives you confidence and fortitude while dealing with the discomforts and inconveniences of treatments and facing the uncertainty surrounding complications and routine checkups.

You are a survivor following completion of treatment. Knowing that you are a survivor gives you a hopeful view of the future while beginning the transition to your "new normal" after illness. You appreciate your resilience while dealing with the challenges of recovery, and you nourish hopeful energy while trying to make your "new normal" an even better one in as many ways as possible.

You are a survivor as you complete recovery and become a long-term survivor. Knowing that you are a survivor gives you hopeful momentum while integrating your past illness into your life today so that you can move beyond illness.

You are a survivor while living with terminal disease. Knowing that you are a survivor gives you power, self-respect, and hope while dealing with progressive disease and end-of-life issues. Knowing that you are a survivor allows you to live until you die.

The term "Survivor" is a helpful and hopeful term, and I encourage its continued use. But, it is only a beginning. "Survivor" only says you are alive; it says nothing about your quality of life. In 1992, I offered an additional term: Healthy Survivor. "A survivor who gets good care and lives as fully as possible is a Healthy Survivor." When you do *anything* in a healthy way, you increase your chances of success and, usually, happiness. Healthy financial planning is a way of managing your monies that leads to a fat checking account for today and savings account for tomorrow. Healthy parenting is a way of raising children that leads to solid kids who enjoy loving relationships with you. And Healthy Survivorship is a way of living with and after illness that helps optimize the outcome in all spheres of your life.

> Healthy Survivorship is determined by *how* you live.

Longer life is definitely an important goal. Yet living to a ripe old age does not automatically make you a Healthy Survivor because it also matters *how* you live. "Health" implies a wholeness of body, mind, and spirit.

You can be a Healthy Survivor no matter how sick you are or how long you live. As a Healthy Survivor, you are able to integrate the reality of your illness into your life during and after treatment, and you treasure what you have for as long as possible, even if treatment can't cure, or even control, your disease. The essence of Healthy Survivorship is that while getting good medical care you are living your life as fully as possible, today, tomorrow, and every single day.

The Miracle of Healing

*W*hen I first got sick, I questioned the tenets that had guided my years of work healing others. It wasn't that I had any doubts about the doctor in whose hands I'd entrusted my newly diagnosed body; it was that I was terrified of the treatments he proposed.

Two days after my oncologist had gently broken the news of my cancer, he stood once again at the side of my hospital bed, this time to share his conclusions about which medicines I would begin receiving after the weekend. I suspect his detailed description was intended not only to keep me well-informed like all his other patients but also to help me feel more in control by talking to me like a fellow physician. Unfortunately, my only contact with these drugs had been during medical school and postgraduate training when I'd feverishly committed to memory their notorious risks. The unintended effect on me of my oncologist's approach was to prompt an ever-more-frightening mind game of "What's the risk of this drug?" When he said, "We are going to use nitrogen mustard," I automatically thought, "Leukemia. Nitrogen mustard causes leukemia. Ding! Correct." When he next said, "Adriamycin," ten years' worth of cobwebs dissolved and my anxiety rose: "heart disease." A split second later, he said, "High-dose prednisone." Being an internist very familiar with the adverse effects of steroids, I began rattling off in my head the list of possible long-term complications: osteoporosis, cataracts, diabetes," only to be interrupted by his pronouncement of the next ingredient to be included in my chemo-cocktail: "Cytoxan." I couldn't remember exactly what the complication was, but I knew it had something to do with the bladder. "Vincristine? Um, nerve damage. Methotrexate? . . ." His prescriptions sounded like a page out of my toxicology textbook.

I'd always nourished and protected my body. Knowing that conventional cancer therapy gave me my best chance of surviving did little to soften the dread that I was about to ruin my body forever. Was I really going to open my veins to these highly toxic chemicals?

The essential question you ask after being diagnosed with a serious medical problem is "How can I get well again?" Your answer, which reflects your beliefs about healing, is critical because *what* you do affects *how* you'll do. And, what you expect affects how you'll feel about what is happening.

It's easy to fall into some common traps when dealing with the shock of a new diagnosis, the discomforts of treatment, the disappointment of medical complications, or the frustration of a slow recovery. Maybe you feel as if your body has failed you by getting sick or that your doctors have failed you if you develop problems during or after treatment. If you have cancer, your confidence that conventional therapies can kill all your cancer cells may be overshadowed by your perception that using these harsh therapies is like using a hammer to kill an ant on a glass window: You fear they will hamper or destroy your body's natural ability to fight your disease and, worse, hurt your body's ability to recover and function normally ever again. And, after hearing from friends, family, the media, and the self-help literature that a positive attitude is critical to healing, you may feel confused about your role in your own healing.

What about the nonphysical dimensions of healing? Maybe your illness has been a blow to your self-esteem, sense of security, optimistic nature, and financial security. Important relationships may be strained. Your faith in God may be tested. In order to achieve wholeness, you may need to heal not just your body but also your emotional, psychological, financial, social, or spiritual selves. How does healing in these areas affect your physical well-being? What does this word—*healing*—even mean?

What does "healing" mean for you?

Healing and Recovering

To heal is to lessen a hurt, repair a breach, and create a sense of completeness. To recover is to regain what's been lost. Ideally, healing will lead to your recovery. Yet, even if complete or partial recovery is not possible, you still can take steps to heal as you face ongoing physical challenges and losses. You may have trouble believing it now, but it is possible to end up even stronger and better than ever in one or many ways.

Knowing that your body responds in healing ways to illness and injury can help calm your fears. Understanding how treatments help your body recover can dispel common myths and misconceptions that lead to confusion, unwise treatment choices, discouragement, or despair. Learning healthy and hopeful ways of thinking about your body's ability to heal, and learning about the role of effective treatments in healing, will help you find the confidence and energy you need to move forward.

> After healing, you may end up stronger and better than ever in one or many ways.

Your Physical Self-Healing Potential

Your body is wired to heal itself. Each instant your body senses threat, mechanisms are automatically set in motion to prevent or minimize damage, and repair any damage that occurs. Then, repair processes continue to work on damaged areas until your body can do no more to help. Knowing that your body is forever working to keep you safe, you may be wondering, "How did I get in this condition? Why can't my body get well by itself?" To answer these questions, let's talk about your body's self-healing potential.

Recovery from injury or illness without the use of medication or procedures is known as "spontaneous healing" or "natural healing." Scrapes, head colds, food poisoning, and innumerable other minor injuries and illnesses usually go away completely over time, leaving you with no trace of the problem. You truly are "as good as new," and your wound or illness can be forgotten. Other times, after healing is completed, you are left with a permanent scar or weakness of some sort. If you sustain a clean cut that goes through all the layers of your skin, you'll be left with a line of a scar. This healing still is "completed" because it is the best your body can do and all repair processes cease. Other scars are on the inside of your body, such as the permanent spot on your chest X ray after you've been treated successfully for certain types of pneumonia. Still other "scars" are microscopic and only apparent as signs, symptoms, or as abnormalities on scans or blood-test results. For example, years after a wrist fracture has healed properly, your wrist may ache in rainy weather even though X rays and a thorough physical exam are completely normal.

What about cancer, diabetes mellitus, and other serious illnesses? Why can't you depend on the self-healing mechanisms of your body to cure you?

The Limits of Your Self-Healing Potential

Your body's normal self-healing abilities have limits. Let's take a closer look at what happens when you get an infection. Minor colds usually don't slow you down too much, and you get better with tincture of time. More significant infections like the flu or a forty-eight-hour stomach virus can make you miserable until your immune system rids you of the invaders. But with serious infections like bacterial pneumonia or meningitis, your body needs the help of antibiotics to dash these harsh germs. The limits of your body's natural ability to heal become obvious when you are infected with organisms that are too virulent and/or numerous for you to expect (or, even hope) to recover without medical intervention.

When talking about healing from cancer rather than from infection, the implications are a bit different by the time you develop symptoms. Your immune system's seek-and-destroy antitumor patrol (called "immune surveillance") is designed to kill incipient tumors before they ever have a chance to become established. On occasion, cancer cells escape this first line of defense. The rogue cells multiply. If they continue to escape detection, malignant cells heap up into tumors and, at some point, may spread to other parts of your body. The reason that some microscopic cancers are eliminated and others grow unabated is not well understood but is under intense investigation by research scientists. Your cancer has to breed *billions* of cells before it can cause you to have any symptoms or be detected by even the most sensitive screening tests. As the number of malignant cells continues to increase, your healthy cells are threatened. Aside from exceptionally rare situations, by the time you are diagnosed with cancer (even if you are diagnosed with an early cancer), your body's *natural* ability to rid itself of malignant cells already has been exceeded.

For some other diseases, the underlying problem is a loss of specific cells that perform a unique and vital function in the body. This loss can be due to toxins, aging, infection, decreased flow of blood (ischemia), the immune system turning against normal cells (autoimmunity), or some as-yet-unknown cause of cell death. The body has no mechanism to replace those lost cells, much as you can't grow a new limb; without these specialized cells, illness is inevitable. For example, the movement disorder characteristic of Parkinson's disease is due to loss of particular brain cells that produce dopamine. In patients with type 1 diabetes, loss of insulin-producing cells causes life-threatening elevations of blood sugar.

Lucky for you, methods have been developed to overcome many of these limits of self-healing. In any health crisis, you can maximize your chance of a good outcome by taking rational action that has been proven to help others in similar circumstances. If your clothes were to catch fire, you'd do best to suppress your urge to run, and, instead, "stop, drop, and roll." In the minutes following a deep cut to a limb, you'd better use a tourniquet to staunch the flow of blood. When you are diagnosed with serious illness, your best response is not to depend on your body alone to get you better but to seek expert medical advice about effective treatments.

Do you think your body can get well without treatment? Whom do you call and what do you do when you are seriously ill?

Setting the Stage for the Miracle of Healing

With your life threatened by disease, you may find yourself wishing for a miracle—a recovery that is awe inspiring and wonderful. Maybe you've always believed in miracles, and hoping for one now is the most natural response in the world. If skeptical before, this is the time when the possibility of a miracle seems worth considering.

I have long been in awe of the miracle of healing. As a physician, I witnessed amazing recoveries of some of my sickest patients. My own recovery from cancer just deepens my confidence of the healing powers of the body. After all, in 1993, when my cancer recurred for the second time, my long-term future looked bleak. Scientific statistics put my life expectancy at about two years. Now, over eleven years later and after five more courses of treatment, I am enjoying a complete remission that began over six years ago. Granted, my treatment courses and recoveries were not easy, and I am now dealing with aftereffects that include energy limitations and an increased potential of various medical problems such as second cancers. But to be alive at this point is a miracle of modern medicine, and my recovery is humbling.

Because of my books and lectures, I get e-mails and calls from patients who've heard my story. They want to know, "What's the secret? How did you beat the terrible odds?" I tell them what I know: Healing is hard work.

Healing miracles do happen. You need to make them happen.

I don't sit in my chair, clasp my hands together, and wait for healing events that defy the laws of nature. I muster my resources—the best that science and technology have to offer me as well as the many factors that nourish healing such as diet, exercise, and a healthy state of mind—to set the stage for my recovery. It's up to you to find out what you can do to help your body heal. It's up to you to do what you have to do to help it happen. As I see it, your physical healing, like the blooming of a carefully tended orchid, is a miracle beyond comprehension that depends on your efforts.

Do you believe in healing miracles? Do you believe you can take steps to help your body heal?

The Role of Treatment

A treatment is a procedure or medicine that will aid your natural healing process when your body is threatened by illness or injury. No matter what medical treatments you receive—surgery, antibiotics, chemotherapy, radiation, immune therapy—*your body* still does the healing, not the treatments. Medical therapies simply expand the limits of your body's self-healing potential, turning the impossible into the possible, and the improbable into the likely.

Say you cut your finger with a sharp knife. If left alone, your wound might get infected and you'd likely be left with an unsightly scar. In contrast, a few well-placed sutures can assist the healing process by holding the two sides of the cut close together. So positioned, your injury easily falls within your body's realm of healing that you'd expect with a more minor cut. Stitches decrease your chance of developing a wound infection and increase the likelihood of a cosmetically acceptable scar. Note that the needle and thread can't heal your wound (suturing a wound in a corpse would not lead to healing); rather, using a needle and thread properly makes it more likely that *your body* will heal your wound completely. In a similar way, draining an abscess or taking antibiotics can convert a serious bacterial infection that might be beyond your body's ability to heal on its own into a problem that your body now can manage with reliability.

Now, let's look at cancer. All conventional anticancer therapies help your body get rid of your malignant cells, making it far more likely that your inborn antitumor mechanisms can regain control. Most standard cancer treatments work by injuring or destroying the offending cells—in this case, your cancer cells. Your body can then destroy any remaining cancer cells, clear away the dead and dying cells (both the cancer cells and the immune cells that are used up in the process), and repair damage to normal cells caused by their encounters with cancer cells and/or cancer therapies. Immune modulators such as interferon and newer cancer therapies such as monoclonal antibodies focus on your body's response to cancer. They boost your innate tumor-killing potential. Effective cancer treatments make it possible (or probable) for your body to heal after developing an otherwise fatal condition.

In cases of illnesses due to malfunction or destruction of vital cells, effective treatments can help compensate for the abnormalities. For instance, various medications and surgical procedures can often diminish the symptoms of Parkinson's disease, and for many patients with diabetes, injections of man-made insulin help keep blood sugar levels in normal or near-normal ranges.

What types of treatments might help your body heal?

The Body Gets the Credit—Who Cares?

You might be wondering why I'm making such a big deal about this distinction between "your body" getting you better and "your treatments" getting you better. I want to dispel a popular myth. A concept that is especially popular in the world of cancer survivorship is that conventional therapies impair or destroy your body's self-healing powers. Although many conventional cancer therapies do, indeed, impair certain aspects of immune function (usually temporarily), when you look at it from the point of view of your *overall* physical healing, every conventional therapy has been proven to help your body's ability to heal from cancer.

Another myth that arises out of the mistaken belief that your therapy does the healing is that the *only* measure that makes a significant difference in your recovery is getting the right prescriptions for medical treatment. This myth encourages people to give little or no effort to measures that might also help your body heal while you are taking the best prescribed therapies. You might mistakenly pay too little attention to eating well, resting well, and getting physical activity.

Here is one more reason why I belabor the point about the body doing the healing: You may feel calmer and more confident if you know that toxic conventional therapies help your body heal even when they make you weaker in the short run. Take a moment to think about the many nonmedical situations where you make something temporarily weaker in the process of repairing it. For instance, a Texas storm caused hail damage to our shingle roof, which was now at risk of developing serious leaks during subsequent storms. We contracted to have the roof repaired while the damage was still relatively minor. In order to fix the problem, the roofers first had to make our home *more* vulnerable by stripping off all the old shingles (which is why they postponed our start date when the forecast predicted rain). As a patient, when my counts are low or I'm feeling sick and tired during cancer treatment, I think about our house in the process of getting a new, sturdy roof. Vulnerability can be a normal part of a successful repair that makes things better in the long run.

> Vulnerability can be a normal part of the healing process.

In what ways are your treatments making you weaker or more vulnerable in the short run? In what ways will your treatments make you stronger and healthier in the long run?

The Disease-Treatment Tightrope

If treatments can get you well when otherwise you wouldn't, what's the problem? Anyone who has taken a powerful antibiotic or signed a consent form for surgery knows that many of today's successful treatments come at a price: In exchange for benefits, you incur risks. Antibiotics that fend off pneumonia or a wound infection may cause an upset stomach or, worse, may trigger a life-threatening allergic reaction. Surgery may repair the injured organ but leave you with an area of numbness or, worse, be complicated by postoperative bleeding or stroke. When the problem is cancer, most treatments tend to be expensive and time-consuming, and they can increase your chance of developing deleterious medical conditions, now or later.

It is possible that your life expectancy is the same with or without treatment, or your disease is expected to respond just as well if treated later as now (an unusual situation in oncology). If this is the case, withholding treatment ("watch and wait" or "wait and see") would preserve your overall quality of life for as long as possible. End-of-life palliative care—care aimed not at cure but at keeping the patient most comfortable—is indicated when the downsides outweigh the upsides of aggressive treatment.

The challenge of determining the optimum treatment for you is like walking a tightrope: If you receive too little medical therapy with the hope of sparing you side effects and aftereffects, you increase your chances of suffering or dying from treatable or curable disease because of undertreatment. If you receive too much therapy in hopes of ensuring a cure, you increase your risk of dying from the treatment (now or later) or surviving with an unacceptably compromised quality of life. In an ideal world, optimum treatment affects only diseased cells, causes few or no side effects, and carries no risk. In the real world, optimal treatment finds the best balance of effectiveness and risks *for you*.

What price might you have to pay to get well? What is likely to happen if you receive too little therapy? Too much therapy?

Physical Healing

Physical healing means returning your body to its pre-illness condition *as much as is possible*. Your physical healing is an active process that is assisted by the effective healing measures you pursue, and continues until your body can do no more to make things better. In many cases, the same medical treatments that can save your life often injure some of your normal tissues, causing side effects and, possibly, complications during your course of therapy, as well as unwanted aftereffects once your treatments are completed. Depending on the particular problem, your physical challenges during and after treatment may be temporary or permanent, obvious or subtle, immediate or delayed.

Rest assured that as soon as your body sustains any treatment-related injury, additional healing processes are set in motion to address it, and these repair processes continue until your healing is as complete as possible. As already mentioned, some survivors end up healthier than ever before. This can happen when their illness acts as a powerful wake-up call, and they abandon unhealthy behaviors. For example, imagine a patient whose light heart attack prompts her to quit smoking. She also adjusts her work schedule and improves her diet, sleep, and exercise regimens. Any decrease in her overall health due to her heart attack is overshadowed by improvements in her lung function, weight, cholesterol, blood-sugar levels, energy, conditioning, and state of mind.

The bad news is that healing may leave you with physical scars of some sort, namely, changes that can lead to symptoms or problems, now or later. The good news is that you are alive, and you are free to choose how you deal with your scars. Your actions and perspective will help determine the overall effect, if any, of these scars on your life.

Physical Healing—Cure

*Cure: You have no detectable sign of disease
and no more chance of your disease coming back
than if you'd never had it.*

In the early 1990s, after being diagnosed with "the big C," I was totally focused on the other "C" word: Cure. I wanted to be cured of my cancer. Who wouldn't? With time, experience, and reflection, my understanding of physical healing after illness evolved and led me toward a more useful focus: being healthy. Although cure is, and always will be, desirable, it is no longer my chief goal. In fact, I don't need to be cured to be healed—even physically healed.

Theoretically speaking, when you are cured of your disease you don't have a single abnormal cell left in your body. From a practical clinical point of view, cure means that you have no detectable disease *and* you have no greater chance of developing your illness again than if you'd never had it. When I sat down and thought about *why* I wanted to be cured—namely, so I could live my life—it was suddenly obvious that cure was not a necessary condition for living a satisfyingly complete life. I don't need for every last cancer cell to be gone to feel well, happy, or fully alive, nor do I need a guarantee that my cancer will never come back once I'm in remission. It was liberating for me to realize that, with my disease well controlled, my life could be at least as wonderful as if I were cured.

Under many common circumstances, people don't feel the need to be cured to be healthy. Would you consider yourself to be *unhealthy* if you had a bad back from an old injury? Certainly, following the accident, you might see yourself as unhealthy during your evaluation and treatment. After that, you would probably move forward, adjusting your life to deal with any back problems that remain. What if your arm were in a cast? What if you had well-controlled hypertension or age-related farsightedness or allergies to cats? In all these cases, your health wouldn't be perfect, but I suspect you'd see yourself as healthy. When I was feeling pretty well during my final round of antibody treatments, someone once said to me, "I'm so sorry you're sick." I answered happily, "I'm not sick! I just have cancer."

> You can feel healthy and get on with your life while your medical problems are being managed with therapy.

When you have a medical problem, you are not sick unless you are sick. You are not dying unless you are dying. You can be healthy even though your back may hurt when you drive for long periods of time, your arm is scrawny from months of being encased in plaster, your blood pressure or blood sugar are controlled only when you take medications, your vision is clear only through glasses, your nose itches and eyes water whenever a cat is nearby, or your CT scans show well-controlled cancer. While your medical problem is being managed with therapy, you can feel healthy and get on with living your life.

Right now, are you sick? Or do you just have a medical problem?

Cancer as a Chronic Disease

Do you see yourself as healthy? If you have cancer, it may be harder than if you have heart disease or diabetes, even if your overall prognosis is actually better. Part of the difficulty may be that, until as recently as the 1960s, newly diagnosed cancer patients faced what felt like a flip of the coin: Either they were going to be cured or they were going to die of cancer. Since then, the development of effective treatments has made cancer one of the most curable and treatable of chronic diseases. Almost ten million Americans today are cancer survivors, and over half of these survivors are cured. Yet, people still tend to think of cancer as a death sentence because many patients have types of cancer that tend to be resistant to the best available treatments, and because too many patients still die of their cancer despite doing everything right.

What is new to cancer healing is the fact that many patients are not cured by their treatments, yet they don't die. Similar to the experience of people with diabetes or rheumatoid arthritis, over one million Americans are now estimated to be living with cancer as a chronic disease. These survivors live for long periods of time dealing with a disease that waxes and wanes or recurs and resolves over and over again. Given the high likelihood of landing on the side of the coin after cancer—living with cancer as a chronic disease—it's outdated to think of cure as the only way to physical healing.

If you have chronic cancer or some other chronic condition, what does modern-day physical healing mean for you? For me, healing is when my body is controlling the growth and spread of my diseased cells. Ideally, you will be able to control your disease with curative treatment. Cure—making this your last episode of this illness—is always desirable when treatment makes this truly possible with acceptable risk. But as you can see from my definition of physical healing, all is not lost when cure is not likely with current treatments. Some effective treatments won't cure you, yet may get your disease into remission or partial remission, or may stabilize or compensate for the abnormalities for long periods of time, thus allowing you to live a long and healthy life.

What does "cure" mean to you? How important is it to you to be cured?

Healed, for Now

For anyone dealing with a disease that tends to recur or is an ongoing condition, thinking of cure as a necessary condition for good health can make things worse. For example, patients who have been diagnosed with

a type of cancer that is very curable today still have to go through treatments and recovery and then wait the specified number of years before
their physicians can say they are cured. To suggest that you are not
healed unless you are cured makes it harder for you to relax about your
health until the requisite number of years has passed. A focus on cure
can make you feel anxious about your health when you are actually
doing well, and this sense of heightened vulnerability often impedes living fully.

For years now, when I've been in remission, I've no longer needed or
even wanted to know if I was cured. It simply didn't make any difference
in the context of the *overall uncertainty* about my future health. Even if I
knew in some magical way that my lymphoma was cured forever, I'd still
be at risk of developing other medical problems. With or without a history of cancer, my future health is uncertain. As long as I'm alive, illness
and injury will be risks, irrespective of my cancer status.

If you're healthy today, you are healthy. If your disease is in remission,
you can feel healed even without a guarantee that every single diseased
cell is destroyed or that your disease won't flare up again, somewhere,
someday. If you are dealing with chronic illness, you can experience a different type of healing, one in which you pursue measures to keep your
disease well controlled while you live your life.

Physical healing: curing disease or controlling disease
and its damaging effects until better remedies come along.

Physical Healing—Repairing Damage

Physical healing after illness also involves repair of your healthy tissues
that were damaged by the disease and its treatment. In cancer patients,
except for targeted therapies (such as Gleevec, a novel treatment that
affects only cancer cells), all standard cancer therapies injure some of
your normal tissues to one degree or another. Your healing is complete
when repair processes cease after doing the most they can do to return
your body to an optimal state. What comprises an optimal outcome
depends on what is physically possible. You can be "as good as new" if

- some normal cells are damaged or killed but then are repaired completely or replaced with healthy new cells (for example, the lining of your gut may be damaged by antibiotics or chemotherapy; after treatments are over, the lining of your gut replenishes itself and works normally), or if
- some of your normal cells are damaged or killed, and are never replaced, but your remaining healthy cells can take over the function of the lost cells for a long time, if not indefinitely (for example, drugs that damage some kidney cells cause the remaining kidney cells to work overtime. Your kidney function can remain normal for years, if not for the rest of your life).

Yet, after complete healing, you might never be "as good as new." This is the case if some of your normal cells have been damaged or killed by your disease or therapy and the remaining healthy cells are unable to take over the lost function. The type and degree of your symptoms or problems depend upon the role played by the involved cells in that organ's functioning. For example, damage to the bladder cells may cause you to need to use the bathroom every one to two hours. Such injury would be inconvenient for the average person and a major problem for a marathon runner. Damage to nerve endings in your fingertips could decrease their sensitivity, a loss that might barely be noticed by the average person but would be career ending to a concert pianist.

Another end result of medical treatment can be that some normal cells are damaged in ways that remain silent for a long period of time but turn up as a new problem when that part of the body is stressed, injured, or undergoes age-related changes. These scenarios still represent "complete physical healing after illness" because it is the best your body can do, and repair processes are no longer involved. A friend of mine was cured of Hodgkin's lymphoma as a young adult after receiving radiation to her lungs. Decades later, she needed surgery involving her chest wall. Postradiation changes invisible to the naked eye interfered with the ability of her skin to heal. She had a long and complicated recovery after her surgical incisions broke down. These examples show how complete healing can leave you at risk of future problems.

The Best Chance of a Good Outcome

While it is only human to want a cure after being diagnosed with serious illness, I have found more peace and happiness in setting my sights on achieving the most complete physical healing possible. Think about it: The best you can do is *the best you can do!* How you go about achieving this goal depends on the medical problems you are facing. In almost all cases, this requires a two-pronged approach of (1) controlling the abnormality that is causing problems and (2) preventing and minimizing detrimental effects caused by the abnormality and your treatments.

How, exactly, do you do this? By using effective treatments that convert major health challenges into more manageable ones. No simple set of specific recommendations can possibly apply to all patients, such as, "Operate and cut it out!" or "Take one gram of vitamin C every morning." Your illness is unique. Even recommendations regarding eating and sleeping are best tailored to you. In order to maximize your healing, find out what measures might help *you,* and what might hurt *you.* Always keep in mind that you are the main actor in your healing; only you can take all the steps necessary to maximize your own personal ability to heal.

You are the main actor in your healing.

Now we are going to shift gears from a theoretical understanding of healing to more specific steps you can take to stack the odds in your favor and set the stage for the miracle of healing in your life. Many varied factors come into play in your healing. Choosing a course of medical treatment is the most important decision you will make, so chapter 6 is devoted to making wise treatment decisions with your physicians. Once your treatment has begun, you can help your treatment work effectively by taking all your medicines and therapies properly.

Is getting the right medical treatment all you can do? No, of course not. You can do more. In the setting of the best available medical therapy, your nutrition, exercise program, sleep habits, and emotional and spiritual health can help stack the odds in your favor. The next few sections will focus on a few specific areas under your control that can affect your physical outcome positively. Always keep in mind that these measures, although important elements of your physical healing, are secondary to therapies aimed directly at your disease. One newly diagnosed cancer patient in my support group got so caught up in figuring out what to do about his diet that he didn't spend time learning about his cancer treatment options and felt overwhelmed when it was time to choose. A heart patient of mine was far more vigilant about reporting changes in her mood to her minister than reporting physical warning signs to me. As a Healthy Survivor, distinguish between therapies that can control your disease and health measures that can help you feel better and improve your condition.

In what ways can you help your body heal?

First, Do No Harm

As a medical student eager to fix my patients' medical problems, I learned from a wise physician that sometimes the best approach is to "hurry up and do nothing!" Dangers can arise when patients feel compelled to do more, trying to ensure a good outcome or speed up the healing process. With the best of intentions, patients take over-the-counter medications or self-prescribe therapies that interfere with their conventional treatments and/or the body's self-healing mechanisms. It happens all the time. A doctor places stitches across a gap in the skin, and then the patient goes home and puts a cream or bandage on the wound that would have healed faster and better if left open. An athlete thinks, "No pain, no gain," and continues his or her rigorous exercise program while fighting a certain type of viral infection, inadvertently increasing the chance of developing heart muscle damage. Many cancer survivors ingest huge dosages of specific supplemental vitamins in the mistaken belief that if a little is necessary for healing, more is better. Unfortunately, such vitamins taken in high doses can affect the blood levels of many types of chemotherapy, and patients can inadvertently increase the toxicity of their cancer treatments or decrease their effectiveness.

First, do no harm! Always confer with your physician as to what non-prescription treatments and supplements might interfere with your body's ability to benefit from your treatments.

First, do no harm!

When the wisest approach is to give your body time to recover from treatment, comfort and hope can be found in the notion that the miracle of healing often requires patience.

Are you doing anything that might interfere with healing?

Nutrition

A Lamborghini is a fast and powerful car. Yet put only one gallon of good-quality gasoline in its tank, and you'll have a very short ride. Put in a full tank of watered-down gas or let the oil run dry, and this superb machine will sputter to a stop. Similarly, your diet can either give you an edge in healing or can hurt you. Food and water are the essential fuels for your body. Especially when the terrain is rough, having enough of the proper fuel is essential to optimum performance. Your body—made up of all the healthy cells that make you who you are (and that can get you better)—needs proper nutrients to perform at all, let alone to perform optimally under stress.

One trap that survivors can fall prey to is "listening to your body." Your body can send out misleading signals. A lack of appetite does not necessarily mean you don't need food. I was nauseated throughout my first course of chemotherapy because today's effective antinausea medications were not yet available. For a long time, I saw mealtime not as a pleasurable social activity but as an unpleasant task that, like having surgery or taking my chemotherapy, took high priority because it could help my body recover. I forced myself to eat healthful foods when I could get them down, and I drank doctor-approved nutritional liquid supplements when I couldn't eat.

As a Healthy Survivor, learn how to optimize your diet for your particular circumstances. For one, your body may need extra calories during and after treatment. Fighting infection or cancer or other disease and repairing treatment-related injury burns lots of calories. Even if you are lying in bed all day, your body may have increased energy needs as if you were running a race.

Your needs for protein, fluids, and certain vitamins and minerals may be increased during treatment and recovery, too. Providing your body the extra-high-quality fuel it needs to get rid of diseased cells, clear out dead and dying cells, fight infections, promote wound healing, and keep your organ systems functioning well (heart beating, lungs breathing, kidneys filtering, and so on) may help you get better. In most cases, being well nourished will help you feel better.

What you eat is one aspect of your health care that is fully under your control. Talk with a registered dietician or someone else on your health-care team about optimizing your nutrition as you go through diagnosis and evaluation, treatment, recovery, and long-term survivorship.

What measures are you taking to optimize what you eat and drink? Who is helping you get the best nutrition?

Circulation

Your circulation—namely your arteries, veins, and lymphatic vessels—is important to healing because it is the supply line to all your cells. A well-functioning circulatory system may assist healing by bringing medications closer to your diseased and injured cells, and by bringing oxygen and nutrients to all your healthy cells that are working overtime to try to control your diseased cells and repair injured ones. Also, good circulation may help healing by carrying away wastes, not only from tissues that are affected by your illness but also from your "cleaning" organs such as your kidneys and liver. You can take steps to improve your circulation. Talk with your health-care team about hydration, medications, and conditioning exercises that can optimize your circulation to all parts of your body. These efforts may help your body control your disease, minimize treatment-related injury, and repair any damage that occurs. Improved circulation may help you feel better while you get better.

What measures are you and your physicians taking to optimize your circulation?

Exercise

To exercise is to use your muscles for health. Exercise affects your hormones, circulation, muscles, bones, heart and lungs, nervous system, and state of mind. Moderate-intensity exercise such as thirty minutes of brisk walking has been shown to improve certain measures of immune function in healthy people. Researchers expect the current studies being done on cancer patients to confirm what already has been shown in patients with other chronic diseases such as heart disease and diabetes: Fitness is associated with improved outcomes and decreased mortality. Numerous studies have shown that moderate-intensity exercise by patients decreases their stress and improves their quality of life. An exercise program tailored for your current medical condition can promote physical changes that enhance the effectiveness of your medical therapies and/or help your body deal with their toxic effects.

Fitness is associated with improved outcomes and quality of life.

It would be a terrible disappointment if you tried to help your situation through exercise and ended up causing a preventable medical problem. Before you start any exercise program —even walking—have it approved by your physician, perhaps in consultation with a physical or exercise therapist. During treatment, your body is subjected to many stresses and may be weakened. You may need to make adjustments and take special precautions. For example, if you have a low red-blood-cell count (anemia), you may need to decrease the intensity of your workout. If you have a low white-blood-cell count, you may need to avoid infection-prone environments and equipment. You may be discouraged from swimming in pools or lakes.

A common trap is to assume that you are too weak, tired, or debilitated to exercise. Almost always, an exercise program can be designed that will accommodate your condition's restrictions. Even if you can't get out of your bed or chair, you can be taught exercises to improve your overall fitness and circulation, making an important difference in your quality of life.

What if you just don't feel up to it? Whenever I don't feel like working out, I remind myself of the overall goal of my treatments: to help me regain my health. I think of exercise in the context of my cancer therapies: If I can willingly roll up my sleeve for intravenous chemotherapy, surely I can make myself go for a brisk walk or perform some other exercise. Fitness is an essential element of good health that is under your control. The added benefit is that exercise is one way for you to regain a sense of control by contributing actively to your care. Talk with your health-care team about an exercise program that can help you improve your sense of well-being during treatment and speed your recovery after completion of treatment.

What exercise are you getting? In addition to your physicians, who can offer you solid advice about setting up a program?

Sleep and Healing

When you turn off the power switch to a motor, everything shuts down and gets quiet. In contrast, when you close your eyes and fall asleep, the physical healing processes of your body continue. Many complex events in your brain and body actually become *more* active during sleep, a time of restoration. If you could hear your healing, the sound would probably be thunderous while you are off in dreamland. Nighttime is when energy stores are restocked, the daily wear and tear on your body is repaired, and the wrinkles of stress are smoothed out. If you want to help your healing, get lots of good-quality sleep!

Chronic sleep deprivation has well-documented adverse effects on overall health. Insomniacs who are otherwise healthy tend to recover more slowly from stressful incidents and are more vulnerable to infections and other illnesses. Beyond the fact that a sleep debt can lead to physical illness, it affects your ability to cope with the stresses of your illness. After a sleepless night, not only do you feel tired and lose motivation, you can also experience mood changes, slowed thinking, decreased reflex time, impaired memory, decreased ability to concentrate, and irritability. Efforts to improve your sleep can activate a positive healing cycle: When you sleep better at night, you are in better shape during the day to tend to existing problems and prevent new problems; by decreasing your overall stress during the day, you sleep better at night, and so on.

One trap that you may fall into is to assume that you are supposed to have trouble sleeping when you are sick, or that such difficulties aren't important enough to mention to your physicians and family. Insomnia—difficulty falling asleep or staying asleep—is a symptom like bleeding or vomiting. Make sure your health-care team knows when you are not sleeping well. If your medications are affecting the parts of your brain that control your ability to sleep, ask your physicians about making medication adjustments that might solve your sleep problem. If physical problems such as pain or urinary frequency are keeping you awake at night, attending to these medical problems takes on added importance. Working through problems that are causing physical, emotional, psychological, or spiritual distress can improve your quality of life during the day and help you sleep at night.

Another trap is not recognizing when sleep deprivation is causing or exacerbating daytime problems other than tiredness. Hopelessness, depression, persistent or worsening pain, difficulty making decisions, poor memory, or tensions at home may be due to or exacerbated by a worsening sleep deficit, and not to a weak spirit, uncontrolled disease, inadequate decision-making skills, dementia, or a failing marriage. Simply put, sleep deprivation can make it difficult, if not impossible, to make wise decisions or deal with the stresses of illness in healthy ways.

Other problems arise from dealing with the practical and emotional strain of needing more sleep. For me, my tiredness and my need for more sleep at night and naps during the day have posed one of the most frustrating and challenging adjustments of my survivorship. During the early years of my illness, I became caught in a vicious cycle of fatigue and poor sleeping. Medications, hormonal changes, and anxiety made it hard to fall asleep or stay asleep. I can't prove that my insidiously progressive sleep debt hurt my physical healing, but I'm sure that it exacerbated the illness-associated stresses. Once I accepted that sleeping is not wasting time and that efforts to improve my sleep could improve my health, I was able to work with my doctors on resolving my sleep difficulties and set up a daily sleep schedule that helped me feel better. Discuss with your health-care team how to optimize your sleep. Try taking a nap in the afternoon. Beware: Too much daytime sleep can interfere with nighttime sleep. Healthy sleep will help you feel better and will help your healing twenty-four hours a day.

What steps are you taking to optimize your sleep?
Have you spoken with your physicians about ways
to optimize your sleep?

Touch

Your skin is your largest organ, providing a physical connection to the outside world. Research has shown that human touch is essential for the normal growth and development of babies. Touch—to touch something, or to be touched—stimulates the nervous system and can cause wide-ranging physical and emotional changes. The right touch at the right time can be healing. A long and gentle bear hug from a caring friend or relative may calm your agitation or comfort you as you grieve. Therapeutic massage may relax your tense muscles, relieve your nausea or pain, and improve local circulation. A sponge bath may cool your anger as well as your fever. A nurse's pat on your back may lessen your sense of fear and loneliness; a friend's hand squeeze may remind you that you are loved and inspire you to carry on. Stroking a soft blanket and resting your head on a fluffy pillow may help you drift off to sleep. At the least, physical connection with others will help you feel better and motivate you to comply with healing therapies. At its greatest, caring touch may help your body heal.

In the setting of serious illness, various obstacles may prevent you from experiencing the benefits of touch. Friends and relatives may withdraw physically, worried about exhausting you or imposing on your privacy. You may inadvertently discourage intimacy with others if your pain or debility makes it impossible to be physically close in exactly the same way you'd always been. If you experience an incident where someone's handshake, hug, or love pat causes you pain, you may become anxious when anyone gets close to you, and others may become fearful of hurting you. Being in the hospital or having your immune system suppressed by treatments may force you to be physically isolated from loved ones. Although not as common in this modern day and age, some people may fear catching noncommunicable diseases.

You have your own special needs for touch—how much touch, what kinds of touch. It's those times when touching and being touched may be most difficult that you may need physical contact the most. Your needs may change over time, too. Try to recognize and satisfy your needs for touch. Just as you wouldn't hesitate to ask for a drink of water, don't hesitate to ask someone to hold your hand. Use the power of touch to help you feel better and get better.

How comfortable are you asking someone to touch you in healing ways?

The Mind-Body Connection

Your mind affects your body. Like diet and exercise, mental state and attitude are factors that affect healing during and after treatment. How can your mind play a positive role in your recovery? Since your attitude and willpower influence your choice of treatments, diet, exercise, and so on, your mind affects your outcome indirectly by affecting what you do. For example, an optimistic attitude may help you complete unpleasant therapies, sleep restfully, comply with a doctor-prescribed exercise program, and eat without benefit of appetite. In these ways and more, your attitude is encouraging you to pursue healing measures that improve your chance of a good outcome.

The mind may have more direct effects, too. All other things being equal (such as receiving exactly the same treatments, eating exactly the same diet, exercising exactly the same amount, and getting exactly the same amount of sleep), many people believe that a strong will to live and a genuine sense of hope seem to help the healing process. It's not uncommon for patients with terminal disease to surprise their health-care team and outlive their prognoses in order to attend a child's wedding or to welcome the birth of a grandchild. People also can learn to use the mind to affect the body in more specific ways. Studies in biofeedback and therapeutic hypnosis have demonstrated that ordinary people can learn to modulate bodily functions that are automatic such as your pulse or blood pressure.

The common trap is thinking that because your mind can *affect* your body, it can *control* your body. Although you can learn to use your mind to lower your pulse by a few beats per minute, you can't use your mind alone to control a racing heartbeat due to ingesting a stimulant such as ephedrine, and you can't use your mind alone to correct a chaotic heart rhythm due to an enlarged heart. As for curing cancer, to put it bluntly, normalizing a mildly abnormal pulse or blood pressure is not the same as controlling the spread of malignant cells.

> Your mind *affects* your body; it does not *control* your body.

If you accept that your mind alone can't control all healing, you might be at risk of another trap: assuming that focusing your mind is not an important element. You might feel that your only responsibility in your healing is getting the right prescriptions and therapies. In some cases that might be so, such as if you had a localized skin cancer. You probably could have a pessimistic outlook and an unhappy demeanor and yet survive your disease because curative surgery would have an overwhelming influence on the outcome. But in many cases of illness, the outcome is far less certain, even when the patient is receiving the best of available treatments aimed at the disease. In these cases, the added benefits of supplementary measures may be just what your body needs to tip your recovery in a positive direction. All the extra steps you can take *in addition to optimal medical therapy*—getting in a healthy state of mind, eating a healthful diet, doing an exercise program, etc.—may significantly influence the ultimate outcome. Even if focusing your mind made no difference in your chances of recovery, you would be maximizing your well-being at little or no cost and may feel better physically and emotionally.

Although you can't expect to "think your disease into remission" through visualization or hypnosis alone, your mind may play an important role in your recovery by helping your nervous, endocrine, circulatory, and immune systems get into a healing mode. Exactly what a "healing mode" entails physiologically is under active investigation. *Chronic* distress, grief, depression, and other untoward mental states are known to affect immune function adversely and appear to impair the body's self-healing potential. Conversely, an overall sense of peacefulness and general happiness may improve your body's immune function and ability to repair damaged tissues. The healing power of your mind, limited though it is, may help the *possible* recovery become more *probable*.

> Your mind plays a major role in alleviating your suffering.

Importantly and without question, your mind plays a major role in alleviating your suffering. Self-relaxation techniques and hypnosis have proven effective in helping control many patients' nausea or pain. Talk therapy has helped alleviate anxiety, guilt, and reactive depression. Your expectations, perceptions, and sense of hope affect your emotional response to illness-related discomforts and inconveniences, losses and disappointments. For instance, interpreting your postoperative pain as a sure sign that your surgery didn't work can put your body into a "giving up" mode, and you may feel sad and depressed. Expecting postoperative pain and seeing it as a marker of being one step closer to getting well can energize you into a "healing" mode and help you feel optimistic and happier.

Engaging the power of the mind to facilitate healing of the body can help you feel better as you get better.

How are you using your mind to help your body?

Joy

"A merry heart doeth good like a medicine." The book of Proverbs teaches that laughter and joy hold great healing powers. Genuine laughter is an involuntary physical response to something you find amusing or ticklish. Joy is a feeling of pleasure or happiness. A number of self-help books mention the health benefits of laughter, and many of the physiological changes are, indeed, good for you. Certainly, a well-timed joke in tense times can trigger a hearty laugh that brings you a moment of much-needed relief. A loved one's graduation or a friend's wedding can make you feel that all is right in the world despite your illness. In all these cases, laughter and joy help you feel better.

What about the link between your happiness and your health? Chronic distress or depression has been associated with a poorer medical outcome from many diseases. As will be discussed in chapter 7, learning about your emotions can help you use your unpleasant feelings in healing ways. In addition, since genuine happiness is associated with health benefits, chapter 10 explores finding happiness when you are sick. Making an effort to find and create moments of happiness may help you feel better and get better.

How are you finding joy in your life now?

Relationships

Healing relationships are essential to Healthy Survivors. By nourishing your hopefulness, confidence, and trust, a healing relationship with your health-care team helps you comply with treatments. You can make your needs known and get your needs tended to as you go through treatment and recovery. Healing relationships outside the medical world are essential to Healthy Survivors, too. Not only will such relationships help you get good care by helping you take good care of yourself between office visits, authentic and loving relationships help you live as fully as possible. Your need to feel heard and loved, and your search for meaning in life are satisfied through your relationships with others.

The converse side is that harmful relationships can interfere with healing. If you don't get along with your doctors or nurses, it becomes harder to get the best care. If family troubles make it difficult to eat or sleep, or keep you in a constant state of emotional turmoil, it is harder to deal with the stresses of treatment and recovery. Whether you are sick or not, dealing with relationships that breed distrust, anger, disappointment, frustration, or ill will makes it tough to enjoy life. I will discuss these healing relationships at greater length in the next chapter on healers.

*How are you developing healing relationships with your
health-care team, family members, friends, and others?
What are you doing about relationships that
are harmful to your healing?*

Stacking the Odds

A perilous trap for patients is to think that if something can help your body heal, it can get you well all by itself. For example, it helps you to realize that nutrition affects your healing; it's dangerous to conclude that proper diet, alone, can cure you. To illustrate this idea, let's look at Lance Armstrong, the cancer survivor who has broken world records in one of the most challenging bicycle races, the Tour de France. Grueling daily practice rides were the key factor that enabled him to win. Other factors helped his stellar performance, too, such as the various dietary regimens he followed. In his autobiography, *It's Not about the Bike*, he describes how he approached his diet with the same scientific rigor as his physical exercise, learning what his body needed for maximum performance when in training and what diet would best energize his body during a race. Armstrong's stunning series of first-place finishes may be attributed in part to the edge offered by his special diets. Even so, he did not depend on diet alone. Had he followed his diet but skipped the physical training on his bike, he wouldn't have had a snowball's chance in the sun of winning the race. In other words, the right diet can help stack the odds in his favor, but proper diet alone can't enable a win.

The key to your recovery is first choosing the best medical therapy *for you* and stacking the odds in your favor by encouraging a healing mode through good nutrition, appropriate exercise, enough sound sleep, a healthy state of mind, and positive emotions. The next chapter will look at the people who can help you find and use the therapies available to help your healing.

Are you getting the most you can out of your medical treatment aimed at your disease? Is your situation the best it can be regarding your diet? Circulation? Exercise? Sleep? Touch? Attitude and state of mind? Joy? Relationships?

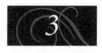

Your Healers

*A*fter being diagnosed with yet another recurrence, all I could think
was "My fairy godmother must be on vacation!"

Who wouldn't like to have a fairy godmother to whisk away medical problems with the wave of a magic wand? Of course, in the real world, you look
to healers—*people* who can teach you about, prescribe, or administer treatments that facilitate your body's healing mechanisms. A wide variety of
people offer therapies for your condition. You need to know who can help
you and how. In our "buyer beware" environment, anyone can call himself a
"healer," so you need to recognize self-proclaimed "healers" who might hurt
you in some way. Just as important is not rejecting flawed healers who *can*
help you in valuable ways. This chapter reviews the people who can help
you get better and feel better, and how to work with them in healing ways.

Helping You "Feel Better" versus
Helping You "Get Better"

To feel better is different from getting better. The best way to feel better *in
the long run* is to control or get rid of the invading organisms, malignant

cells, or whatever abnormality is threatening your health. Even if you feel perfectly fine right now, you may need surgery, antibiotics, blood-pressure medicines, hormones, or chemotherapy. Unfortunately, many effective treatments can make you *feel worse* in one way or another while they are helping your body *get better*. Naturally, you want to feel better. But, when recovery is possible with effective treatment, getting better in the long run is more important than feeling good in the short run.

It is a tempting trap to assume that someone who can make you feel better is helping you get better. Sometimes, nothing could be further from the truth. For example, if you have belly pain due to a swollen appendix that is about to burst, a "healer" could give you morphine, and you would feel better as your appendix ruptures. So, too, a family member can make you feel better by agreeing with your assessment that a worrisome symptom can be ignored, even though immediate medical attention is needed. Smooth-talking con artists can make you feel better by assuring you that their pills will help you, even though the proposed treatment has never been proven effective (or, worse, has been proven harmful). If your fears are tamed and confidence is bolstered, you will feel better emotionally and, possibly, physically. Your body may be shifted into a healing mode, too, but while you seem better in the short run, you may be interfering with the effectiveness of your medical therapies or risking complications.

Feeling better is not the same as getting better.

Feeling better is good, as long as you are also getting better. Your doctors, nurses, and other healers should be doing everything possible to help you feel as well as possible while getting you well. Work with your health-care team to make treatment as smooth as possible. If you have rough days, try focusing on the expected benefit: getting better.

What measures are you taking to get better? Which of these might make you feel worse before they get you better? What measures are you taking to feel better while getting better?

Your Team of Healers

Healers include a variety of medical professionals who contribute to your physical recovery—physicians, nurses, and allied health professionals such as dieticians, physical therapists, and social workers. Friends, family, acquaintances, and even strangers also play important roles in your healing. Family members may bring you nourishing food, friends may run errands or drive you to treatment clinics, and acquaintances may care for your children so you can rest. People you'll never meet also are part of your healing circle: researchers working to find safer and more effective therapies; patient advocates providing information and support; the federal government and the National Institutes of Health developing and funding programs that benefit patients; and philanthropists contributing money to disease-specific funds. All these people are committed to helping make progress in medical care—and your care—a reality.

You have to be in the right place at the right time and do the right things to help their treatments work their wonders. Consequently, establishing and nourishing healing alliances with your doctors, nurses, and other health-care professionals is an essential step to becoming a Healthy Survivor. To do so, you need to have realistic expectations of how each healer can and cannot help you. Just as you wouldn't expect

Without your help, your healers can't perform modern-day miracles.

your plumber to fix the electrical wiring in your fuse box, don't expect your family physician to advise you on the subtleties of sophisticated technologies or treatments he or she has never prescribed. My top-notch internist couldn't tell me which combination chemotherapy would be best for treating my lymphoma. Conversely, don't expect too little, or you'll miss out on opportunities for members of your health-care team to prevent and treat problems. When going through my chemotherapy, I *could* turn to my internist for symptoms and problems that developed during and after my cancer treatments, such as sleep difficulties, respiratory infections, emotional distress, and practical concerns about work and home.

Healers are the link between you and treatments. You play a huge role in making sure your healers provide you access to the best medical care. Ideally, you always receive optimum medical treatments from caring experts. In the real world, the two don't always go together, so keep in mind the distinction between *the treatments* a healer can offer you and *the relationship* within which his or her treatments are offered. A particular doctor may be a certified jerk when it comes to breaking bad news, but you'd be making a mistake to conclude that *the treatment* he or she is recommending is a bad choice. Similarly, if a particular physician is comforting and encouraging but has almost no experience treating patients with your disease, you'd be taking a risk putting all your confidence in his or her treatment recommendations without getting a second opinion. Receiving the best treatment is the top priority.

To get the best of both worlds—the best treatments and the best healers—you may need to be flexible, adjusting your expectations about each of your healers and finding a *team* of experts and support people who, together, satisfy your needs. A friend of mine travels five hundred miles to consult with one particular specialist whenever a major change in her condition prompts a reevaluation of her treatment plan. Why? Because he has a special interest in her particular disease, and he does a better job helping her weigh her various options than the specialist who practices close to her home. The consulting doctor confers with her local doctor and, once a course of treatment has been laid out, my friend returns home for all her treatments. She likes and trusts her local doctor who does a great job following her progress throughout treatment and recovery. And if she needs more detailed explanations or a little tenderness during the course of her treatments, she talks with her nurses, social workers, and her support group.

Sir Francis Peabody inspires generations of healers with the aphorism "Cure as often as possible and comfort always." What follows is a brief look at the individual members of your healing team and the unique services each of them offers you, so you can turn to the right people for the right job in the right way. Ultimately, it's up to you to assemble the best possible team of healers and work with them so they can cure you, whenever possible, and comfort always.

Who are the members of your healing team?

Specialists

Physicians are in the unique and powerful position of providing you access to modern medicine. They, and only they, can prescribe scientifically proven therapies and make sure that your treatments are as safe and effective as possible. A board-certified specialist is the physician who can find out and explain to you exactly what is happening with your disease and what can be done to control or cure it. When your problem is cancer, an oncologist is the key player on your healing team. When kidney disease, a nephrologist. Heart disease, a cardiologist. In most cases, he or she calls the shots regarding your evaluation, treatment, and follow-up, even when nurses, technicians, and other physicians are delivering most or all of your actual care.

In a perfect world, the specialist you are seeing is all-knowing and up-to-date, always available, confident, unhurried, calm, inspiring, entertaining, spiritual, or whatever personal approach makes you feel most reassured. Unfortunately, physicians can fall short in one or another area, so the essential question is "What do you *need* from your specialist, and what do you *want*?" First and foremost, you *need* a physician who is skilled in evaluating and treating people like you with diseases like yours. Second, you need your specialist to be available when you have medical issues that require his or her input. If you develop symptoms or a new lump, it doesn't do you any good to schedule an appointment with a top expert whose first opening for a new patient is three months away. If you want your routine care to be overseen by a particular specialist who happens to lecture internationally and is out of the office six months of the year, you're setting yourself up to be unhappy by choosing such a physician to be your primary doctor for the care of your disease. Third, you need to be able to communicate. You need to understand what your physician is asking you and telling you, and you need your physician to understand what you are saying.

> It's up to you to assemble the best possible team of healers and work with them.

If you are fortunate, you and your specialist enjoy an instant chemistry at your first meeting. Don't be surprised or discouraged if that's not the case. As with most long-term important relationships, good rapport and mutual trust may develop and deepen only over time. If the specialist is well qualified but the two of you are not communicating well, it may help to have a family member or friend accompany you to your first few doctor visits. Your companion can help you understand what your physician is saying and clarify your questions and concerns to your doctor. Or, you could meet with a social worker to help you talk with and understand your doctor better. In this way, you are giving your relationship with the specialist a chance to work so you can benefit long-term from his or her care. As long as you have something to gain from a particular specialist's expertise or treatment, it is worth the effort. If you still can't make the relationship work in healing ways, it is time to switch doctors.

What do you want *from your doctor? What do you* need? *Who can help you get the most out of your first few visits?*

Qualified Specialists

I wish I could give you unreserved reassurance that as long as you are seeing a board-certified medical doctor, you can feel confident that you are getting good advice and care. But I can't. What I can do is help you avoid potential pitfalls and increase your chances of developing healthy relationships with good-quality healers.

It sounds obvious, but keep in mind that your physicians can only prescribe available treatments. I don't begrudge my oncologist my needle stick troubles from having received caustic chemotherapy through the veins of my hands instead of through a port (a device used to administer drugs directly into the large veins near the heart) any more than I begrudge my mother for not taking me home from the hospital in a car seat after I was born. Child car seats weren't used in the 1950s, and infusion ports weren't being used routinely when I was diagnosed because they were so new. The problem was not that my physicians prescribed inferior treatment but that the science and technology had to catch up with the medicine. Feeling anger or regret about my scarred veins would hurt me by weakening my confidence in an excellent doctor who deserves my trust and by causing me to have lingering bad feelings about something that can't be changed. The lesson is that you and your doctors are doing your best with what is available when you need treatment.

Patients hurt themselves when they put unrealistic demands on everyone and expect everything to go smoothly. Medicine is an art as well as a science. Of course I want everything to go perfectly when I am sick! But, miscommunications and unintended consequences happen in the best of situations. As long as a snafu doesn't indicate incompetence, I do better to roll with the punches and stay focused on getting well. For example, the best phlebotomist at my oncologist's office usually gets enough blood with the first stick, but not always. I still let her draw my blood. As another example, when my scans in 1992 showed a new recurrence of cancer, my previous scans were pulled out and reviewed again. In retrospect, the films described as "within normal limits" showed subtle signs of early recurrent cancer. This happens all the time: An innocent-appearing ache, fever, or change in a blood test doesn't cause much worry but, in time, turns out to be the beginning of a serious problem. As a Healthy Survivor, what should you do? Once I found out that my earlier films had been misread as normal, I could have refused to let the same radiologist ever look at my films again. That would have hurt me by depriving me of the services of a superb radiologist. I could have harbored feelings of anger, distrust, or disappointment, but these feelings would have only pulled me down. If I sound too forgiving, think about when you are trying to solve a puzzle or mystery: Don't clues always appear more obvious after you know the answer or conclusion? A certain rate of false positives and false negatives is unavoidable, especially with test results that depend on the reader's judgment.

Highly qualified and honorable physicians do the best they can with an imperfect art. If your doctors aren't solving your problem easily, you may, indeed, do best to get a second opinion or switch doctors. Sticking with incompetent doctors is the worst thing you could do. But don't abandon good physicians who are prescribing the safest and most reliable route to an effective treatment, a route that often involves a series of tests and treatments. Don't judge harshly when your physician misses a clue or a solution that is clear to a consulting doctor who has the advantage of additional information. As long as you are getting good care, it helps you to accept the limits of medicine and focus on what you can gain from your healers. Look forward and work together with your health-care team to make things better.

How do you feel when you learn that a treatment you received has been replaced by a treatment that is safer and/or more effective?

Bad Apples

While I was going through evaluation and treatment, it upset me when people would talk about the "bad apples" in medicine. Anxiety and distrust grow when you read in the media about episodes of patients' rights being violated, a researcher who fudged data, a drug-addicted or morally corrupt doctor, or the problem of unscrupulous doctors accepting kickbacks for ordering certain tests or prescribing specific drugs. Conspiracy theories about the suppression of cancer cures by money-mongering physicians and pharmaceutical companies are frightening when you are trying to decide what to do about your cancer. What is true? Whom can you trust? Should you even be talking about these things now?

Bad apples in medicine are bad apples. No profession—even those dedicated to the moral life—is immune to harboring people who are corrupt. If talking about these issues helps you get good care and live fully, then go ahead and talk about them. When you are a vulnerable patient, talking about the grand problems in medicine or the exceptional corrupt practitioners can make it hard for you to prepare for the challenges ahead. Such discussions can fuel skepticism of the people and system that can help you. I'm not saying you should ignore these problems. I'm saying that when you are sick, you might do better to delay thinking about them until you are well again.

As a cancer patient, it's been easy for me to ignore stories about the bad apples in medicine. I have known the medical world as an insider and have had every reason to trust my physicians and the treatments they were prescribing. In general, doctors are devoted to helping their patients, even those who don't have the best bedside manner. Instead of spending your energy fighting the system, try to work with the system and put together a health-care team that can help you take advantage of what science has to offer.

How do you handle it when you hear a horror story about physicians?

Choosing Your Specialist

My total confidence in my health-care team made it easier for me to deal with the uncertainty and discomforts accompanying my illness. This confidence was built on firsthand knowledge that my oncologist's advice was up-to-date and that he cared about me. If you don't have an ongoing relationship with a specialist before your diagnosis, affirmative answers to the questions below suggest that the specialist being considered could be a good match for you.

Tips for Finding a Good Match

- Is this doctor knowledgeable and experienced in the treatment of my disease?
- Is this doctor available to see me?
- Can I understand this doctor's explanations or advice? If not, do I have someone who can help me understand what he or she is saying?
- Do I trust this doctor to have my best interests in mind?
- Does this doctor treat me with respect and understanding?

- Does this doctor nourish realistic hope?
- Are this doctor's services affordable?

Concerns about highly respected specialists can arise when they were on top of their game ten, twenty, or more years ago, and they haven't kept up with medical advances or they are busy caring for patients eighteen hours a day, leaving little time for studying. Some physicians get ingrained in their old ways of doing things as they near the end of their careers.

A consequence of the explosion of medical information is that physicians, even those who read their medical journals and attend continuing medical-education courses, can't possibly stay up-to-date regarding all the intricacies of diagnosis and treatment for every single disease or problem that falls under the umbrella of their specialty. Consequently, some specialists have become further specialized within their field, such as cardiologists who mainly see patients with abnormal heart rhythms and oncologists who mainly see patients with one particular type of cancer. It takes time for information shared at specialty meetings to filter down, so, for instance, general oncologists might not be as up-to-date regarding information about rare types of cancer as a clinical researcher whose practice is devoted to patients with that particular cancer. Given that medical treatments are changing rapidly in some areas, if you want to be offered the most effective and/or safest treatments you may need to be evaluated by a specialist who is up-to-date regarding the treatment of your specific disease, often just for a one-time consultation.

In general, you compromise your care when you lean on your specialist for all your general medical needs. Highly specialized doctors often won't (or can't) diagnose or treat conditions that fall outside their area of expertise, and their offices are not set up for this kind of care. My oncologist is board certified in internal medicine as well as oncology, but he spends all his time treating cancer. He is not the right doctor to be tending to his patients' hypertension, diabetes, hormone problems, or even routine cancer screening. It is in your best interest to see the right doctors for each of your medical concerns and keep all your doctors informed about what everyone else is doing.

Another potential problem you can avoid is that of your healer's bias.

Doctors tend to recommend what they know best. When various good treatments are available, surgeons tend to recommend a surgical approach while internists might be more inclined to recommend an equally effective nonsurgical treatment for the same condition. "Transplanters" (doctors who perform bone-marrow and stem-cell transplants) tend to recommend transplant more readily than oncologists who have never performed this technology. Just knowing a doctor's bias helps you assess his or her recommendations.

The potential problem of bias also applies to individuals. Physicians who have seen horrible outcomes of a new procedure might discourage it while physicians who have seen dying patients rescued by the same procedure may be more enthusiastic. Physicians who have been wrongfully sued by patients with bad outcomes often become overly cautious in the treatments they recommend and overaggressive in the follow-up tests they order, practicing so-called "defensive medicine." Being aware is the first step to avoiding potential problems of bias.

If your condition doesn't require urgent treatment, one of the most efficient and safe ways to be sure of your options is to obtain a second or third opinion. If possible, seek out a physician who specializes in your exact disease or problem (or as close as possible), preferably a specialist with a different bias than your original doctor. I intentionally sought out the opinion of clinical researchers, transplanters, as well as lymphoma specialists who were not affiliated with research or transplant centers. Seeking the opinions of others physicians in no way jeopardizes your relationship with your primary physician and does not indicate a desire to leave that relationship. My oncologist treats all kinds of cancer, and he has been the primary person caring for me since my diagnosis. Throughout, he has consulted with and helped me obtain second opinions from lymphoma specialists across the country, including researchers who have been on the cutting edge of lymphoma care. As will be discussed in chapter 6, obtaining second opinions is a good way to obtain useful information for making wise decisions about your medical care.

One way to know if you are getting up-to-date advice is to do some research yourself or with the help of a knowledgeable friend or family member. Reputable organizations have Web sites and trained counselors to help you learn about your disease and your treatment options. One downside to this approach is that the process can be frustrating, overwhelming, and time-consuming, none of which helps you while you are adjusting to your diagnosis. More important, the notion of doing your own research brings to mind the aphorism "A little knowledge can be a dangerous thing." Your crash medical course may give you a misguided sense that you know enough about your disease and treatment to know what's best for you. This hurts you when it keeps you from following the wise advice of your physician, who is far more experienced in the subtleties and complexities of your condition and treatment choices. The best way to use your newfound knowledge is to help nourish a healing alliance with your health-care team and to help guide your physician to the best care for you.

Nourish healing alliances with the members of your health-care team.

One important aspect of healing alliances is that your physician understands and respects your philosophical approach to your health. If you want a chance at cure no matter what the risks, you can't get good care from a physician who, because he or she feels it is the wrong decision for you, won't tell you about available options that offer only a slim chance at cure. Nor would you want a doctor who won't support your desire to enter a clinical trial, receive treatment at a major medical center far from home, or use a drug under compassionate-use guidelines. Similarly, if you tend to be risk averse, you may not want to be cared for by a doctor who is always the first on the block to try new treatments or who leans toward the most aggressive treatment regimen whenever faced with two or more comparable options.

Your specialist doesn't need to have the same style or philosophical approach as you, but he or she needs to understand your attitudes, needs, hopes, and desires. You need a physician who *respects* your philosophy about treating your illness and is *committed to working as a team* with you toward common goals in your care. This is more important than finding someone who shares your philosophy because, over time, your philosophy may change.

Take the time to check your specialist's credentials with your local medical society and the national specialty board registry. Find out about a prospective doctor's reputation by asking around. If doctors you've known and trusted for a long time recommend other specialists, or they hesitate to endorse someone or talk in vague generalities, find out more about the specialist you were planning on seeing. Other patients can give you useful feedback on their doctor's style, too, but these opinions don't carry the same weight as those of professionals in the know.

Make sure you can communicate well with your doctors. Choose a doctor who listens to your concerns and responds to your questions. If you have to, teach him or her how to listen! A friend told me how her brilliant physician missed making a timely diagnosis of low thyroid for the simple reason that he wasn't listening to her. Every time she started to explain her persistent symptoms and lingering concerns, her doctor kept stopping her with

Remember: You have a right to good care.

more questions. Taking a direct approach, she said, "If you let me talk uninterrupted, I guarantee that I'll explain myself in less than ninety seconds!" What could her doctor do but listen? When she was done less than two minutes later, he said, "You are right," and their communication opened up.

When you are sick, you feel vulnerable and dependent. You may not want to chance offending your physician by complaining or questioning something being done. To get good care, you need to voice your concerns. Take advantage of the resources, many of which are free, available to teach you how to communicate well with your physicians and advocate for yourself. Create and nourish healing alliances with well-qualified specialists who can link you with the best treatments for you. Make the most of your visits and your relationships.

How well do you communicate with your physicians? What will you do if you feel that you are not being heard, your questions are not being answered, or you are not being given the time and attention you need?

Nurses and Physician Assistants

Nurses and physician assistants (PAs) are medical professionals who are trained to administer science-based medical therapies and comfort measures. They are the ones you may see the longest and most often once your treatments begin. These people are not your doctor's secretaries or technicians who merely administer your treatments; they are highly skilled and knowledgeable professionals. They are in a unique position to link you to treatments and support that can help and to get you through your treatments as safely and comfortably as possible.

Physician assistants are not the same as nurses. Their respective training is different, and only PAs can perform routine care and evaluate and write prescriptions for minor problems and side effects. I've grouped them together here because both nurses and PAs administer treatments and act as your vital link to your doctors. For the rest of this section, everything I say about nurses applies to PAs, too.

Nurses can reinforce and supplement your doctors' explanations, advice, comfort, and inspiration, as well as inform your doctors when, in the course of their evaluation or delivery of treatment, they detect a problem that needs attention. Take advantage of the knowledge, skill, experience, and influence of your nurses.

Keep Your Nurses and Physician Assistants Informed About
- your needs as a patient;
- *ALL* signs and symptoms of possible medical problems, including difficulties with eating, sleeping, and mood;
- difficulties with your medications or home medical equipment;
- difficulties with the nonmedical aspects of your care (transportation, family stress, financial concerns, spiritual crises); and
- communication problems with your physician.

Your nurses can't know what is "best" for you unless you tell them. Make your preferences clear from the beginning so that they can make every effort to honor them. If you would feel more relaxed if they called you by your first name, tell them. If you would feel more confident and dignified if they used your proper name, ask them to call you "Mr.

Smith," and not "Bob" or "honey." There is no "right" or "wrong" way to address patients, only a best way for you. Let your nurses know of any special needs, such as your need for early-morning appointments or for a blanket when you are waiting in a cold room. Tell them up front how much you want to know about your condition, and how much you want to be involved in the medical aspects of your care. Some patients want to know nothing more than where they need to be and when. Other patients want detailed explanations and copies of every test result ever done, and that's fine, too. Just let the nurses know before your visit. This way, they can schedule adequate time for your visit, and they won't be hit with a list of twenty questions or the time-consuming task of copying your test results while other patients are kept waiting.

Nurses are the gatekeepers: They determine who talks with the physicians. This is a good thing for you! They are not trying to keep you away from your physicians or trying to "protect" the physicians from your calls or problems. If your doctors took every call from every patient, they would not be able to be doctors. By talking to your nurse, you get the timeliest answers to your questions and problems. For routine matters, nurses can give you expert advice right away because they are used to dealing with patients going through treatments similar to, if not exactly like, yours. And, as long as you give them an accurate account of your problem, they usually know whether to get your doctor right away, send you to the office or emergency room, or tell you what to do while waiting for their call back with the doctor's answers (or a call back from your doctor).

After a doctor's call or visit, take advantage of your nurse's ability to continue your care where your doctor left off. Your nurse often can give you answers and insights you didn't or couldn't get from your physicians. You may have felt uncomfortable mentioning to your doctor that you are having trouble sleeping or that you are feeling blue. Maybe you've tried talking to your doctor about your lack of sexual drive, but he or she gets fidgety and changes the topic. Or, whenever you ask your doctor, "How bad is it?" he or she answers by talking about treatment options and won't give you a direct answer. For whatever reason, if you have still have questions or concerns after talking with your doctor, talk with your nurses. They can help you get *all* your questions and concerns answered to your satisfaction. They can help prevent or repair miscommunications with your doctors, too.

If you need clarification of information that was shared during your visit with your doctor, don't hesitate to ask your nurse, but understand that he or she can help you only *after* having a chance to review your chart or talk with your doctor. Since every time your nurse takes a phone call, he or she is pulled away from caring for another patient—someone just like you—gather all your information and questions before you call.

You are the central player of the health-care team that can get you better. Be a team player.

Don't hesitate to call if you need help, but if at all possible, try to make one call instead of two, three, or more per day.

Don't struggle with the technical and non-medical aspects of your care, either. Your nurse may be able to help if you are having problems with your infusion pump, the pharmacist who fills your prescriptions, your children's response to your illness, or your medical bills. Even when nurses can't solve all your problems themselves, they usually know who can help you. And when they know that you are dealing with these other issues, your entire health-care team can understand you better and take good care of you.

If you feel angry, disappointed, frustrated, or vulnerable when dealing with your nurses, it is important to determine why and resolve any problems. Make sure that you are not misdirecting your anger. It is not uncommon for patients to unleash anger at their nurses when they really feel angry at the diseased cells creating havoc in their life or at the doctors who made them wait two hours for their appointment before rushing them through a five-minute visit. Nurses are trained to deal with patients' anger, but they are still people with feelings and limits.

Last, keep in mind that you are in the medical office only during your appointments; your nurses are there every working day. If they talk to you in anything other than a professional and caring manner, or if they seem incompetent in any way, you need to talk with the offending nurses. If that doesn't solve the problem, or if you can't talk with them, let your doctor know. Your doctor *needs* to know! Oftentimes, problems can be resolved easily. Occasionally, you may need to be cared for by different nurses, when this is an option. If your nurses all treat you well, but you hear them laughing among themselves at the nursing station or in the break room, this is not a show of disrespect or uncaring about the gravity of your situation. Telling a joke or sharing stories about their weekend escapades while they are preparing your medicines or eating lunch recharges their emotional batteries so that they can care for you with patience, focus, and hope.

How well are you using your nurses and physician assistants to get good care?

Allied Health Professionals

Although your medical doctors are the key players in diagnosing and guiding treatment for your medical problems, you may benefit from special expertise and services offered by allied health professionals—social workers, dieticians, clergy, physical therapists, speech therapists, occupational therapists, massage therapists, acupuncturists, and many other professionals. These health specialists may be able to give you advice or administer an ancillary treatment that may make all the difference in the world as you go through treatment and recovery. For example, a nutritional counselor has the time and expertise to help you nourish your body while it is under stress. Or, as another example, a psychologist has the expertise to diagnose an anxiety disorder or one of the many types of depression. Proper treatment can help you eat and sleep well, which helps rejuvenate your body, which helps your body recover.

Discuss all your discomforts and hardships in detail with your healthcare team, and ask if a referral to an allied health professional might be useful. Better yet, don't wait for problems to develop. Ask about any consultations that might help prevent or minimize future problems that you are likely to develop.

*What problems or concerns do you have that might benefit
from the expertise of an allied health professional?*

Support Volunteers and Support Groups

Unlike your physicians, nurses, and allied health professionals, other members of your healing circle don't have to have strings of letters after their names to assist you. Friends, family members, and health-care volunteers and support group facilitators and members can provide invaluable information and assistance. A family member can set up a phone network so your friends and other relatives can remain informed of your status without your having to talk to so many people. Close family and friends may do some of the health research and take on your previous home responsibilities.

But your innermost circle of supporters needs help, too. Ease the overall demands in your life by allowing volunteers to make meals for your family, do your laundry, or carpool your children. Make hard times a little easier by accepting the companionship of other people who are eager to accompany you to treatments or checkups. The energy you might have wasted on worry is now available for something more productive or pleasurable, and hence, healing. Having a broad support team keeps any one friend or family member from being overburdened.

Special emphasis must be given to a potential fountain of healing: support groups. A good support group has been shown to ease particpants' suffering and improve their quality of life. Ongoing research is following up on earlier studies that suggest that participation in a support group may improve medical outcome, too. For three of the eight years I was in and out of treatment, I relished going to the one place where having cancer was normal, yet the focus was not on my treatments but on *living my life*. At group meetings, I was understood and comforted in ways that were only possible with people who were dealing with similar discomforts and stresses. In their company, I often laughed more than I cried, and what tears I shed were healing because everyone absorbed them, patiently and lovingly, instead of urging me to stifle my sadness. Despite generally excellent communication between me and my husband, it was only at support group that certain fears and misconceptions surfaced, lead- **Support groups** ing to insights that helped my husband help me, and **can be a haven of** me him. In unique and powerful ways, my support group helped me become a Healthy Survivor. And **hope and joy.** you can stop going when you no longer find it a benefit.

Nowadays, you have a wide choice of support groups, including telephone and online groups. (See appendix VI.) Support groups are not for everyone and quality can vary, even from meeting to meeting of the same group. Given the low cost of trying a group once or twice, don't miss discovering what could be for you a haven of hope and joy in difficult times.

Who makes up your current support team? Whom would you like to add to your support team? Which support groups have you tried?

Clergy

Clergy are special healers because the tools of their trade are words and rituals that address the great mysteries of life. While doctors and nurses are helping you deal with *what* is happening to your body and what to do about it, clergy can help you deal with *why* this is happening and the meaning of it all. They can help you tap into your inner (sometimes, hidden) resources of calm, patience, courage, and strength. As will be discussed in later chapters, faith is a different type of "knowing" than the "knowing" that is achieved through well-executed scientific experiments. Clergy can help you find or strengthen your spiritual faith. If you don't belong to any organized religion or believe in God, many clergy still can help you deal with your existential questions such as "Why me?" "What is the meaning of this illness?" "What is the meaning of my life?"

Some people fear that if they need spiritual guidance, they must be dying. That is not the case. The experience and wisdom of a clergyperson may be just what you need to adjust to your diagnosis, make wise treatment decisions with your physicians, get through your treatments, or nourish your recovery whether your prognosis is dismal or rosy. Clergy may be able to help you find a perspective on your situation that helps you live as fully as possible and even grow through it all.

One of the most dangerous traps is when people feel forced to choose: "Either I trust science or I put my faith in God." Science and faith are two separate aspects of dealing with illness that can work hand in hand. Science allows you to take advantage of what is known; faith can help you deal with the mysteries and uncertainties that remain. When faith helps you get good care and feel whole, faith and science complement each other and are healing.

Another problem is when people push you toward a type of faith that upsets you in some way or keeps you from getting good medical care. This can occur when your medical diagnosis invites others' testimonies of faith, in much the way a woman's pregnant shape invites unsolicited tummy pats and inappropriately intimate questions. Your faith is *your* faith. If you are not sure and want to explore if faith might help you with your difficult questions and through these uncertain times, clergy can guide you in your spiritual journey. Exploring these questions in a safe place with others can help you find what is uniquely right for you at this time.

Who can help you with your spiritual questions and concerns?

Access

Not everyone has equal access to modern medical care. Sad, but true. I can only begin to even imagine how it feels if you don't have good medical insurance or you are dealing with other restrictions that make it harder to obtain the care you need. I've been fortunate to have good medical insurance and access to whatever treatment I've needed. Yet this luxury has not blinded me to the current crisis in health-care insurance and distribution of services. I've been listening as experts in the media and various authors and politicians argue about the theoretical causes and potential solutions to the economic health-care crisis faced by millions of

Americans. Through my advocacy work, the heart-wrenching problems of real patients without access to available care have been brought home.

Efforts to improve access are vital, but you need medical care *now*. Today. How can you get the best care possible in our current medical system given your financial situation? For the moment, forget about how it might have been if you had better insurance, made more money, or lived in a country where access was universal and all care was first-rate. Instead, focus your attention on how you can get the best care today in your health-care system as it exists today.

Just as learning about your treatment choices helps you make wise decisions, learning about all your options for access to health care helps you get good care. Take advantage of the experiences and efforts of other patients who have been in your shoes. Dedicated individuals and organizations have put together valuable resources to help patients who are dealing with financial constraints. Find out about the many local and national resources available to help you get the most for your money and to get financial and emotional support (see list below).

You deserve good medical care. Make sure the staff at your physician's office knows about your financial situation.

Resources to Assist with Your Access to Care

- National organizations for your disease, such as the American Cancer Society or the National Multiple Sclerosis Society
- Local chapters of disease-specific organizations
- Social-service department of your local hospital
- Community-service organizations
- Religious organizations and communities
- Local public-assistance office
- Illness support groups such as the Wellness Communities and Gilda's Clubs
- Work and school organizations
- Pharmaceutical companies that offer free or reduced-cost drugs to those in financial need
- Your state's insurance and welfare departments
- A financial planner experienced in health care
- An attorney experienced in health care

Your illness may be very expensive, even when your treatments are covered by insurance. You may have too many assets to qualify for public financial support yet be struggling with rising bills and illness-related loss of income. Accepting financial assistance or free services may be difficult for you, especially if you've always been independent. But doing so allows you to better focus your energy on getting well.

Does your health-care team know about your financial situation? Who is helping you find out about financial resources available to you?

Being an Effective Patient

Your illness is *your* illness. Responsibility for getting good care rests in *your* hands. You can get good care and increase the opportunities for joy by being an effective patient. What does it mean to be an effective patient? It means doing what you need to do to help get the intended or hoped-for result.

Effective patients: patients who do what they need to do to help get the intended or hoped for result.

Ways to Be an Effective Patient
- Help your health-care team with your evaluation.
- Work as a team to plan a course of treatment.
- Comply with all their advice during and after treatment.
- Be tuned in to all potential problems or early problems.
- Report potential problems to your health-care team.
- Ensure that your health-care team responds appropriately to your problems and concerns.

Health-care professionals violate your privacy for a noble end: to help you get well. Your doctors and nurses ask you how many bowel movements you have each day and how many alcoholic drinks you consume. I have asked these valuable questions to thousands of my patients. Yet these repeated invasions of privacy exact a price. I know. When I was being restaged to evaluate my first recurrence, the radiologist with whom I had worked for many years explained what he would be doing and looking for on the planned sonogram. Then he politely announced that he would wait outside while I changed into a gown. I said, "Don't bother leaving, Paul. Everyone else has seen me naked this week, why shouldn't you?"

Let's face it: The doctor-patient relationship is unequal, and always will be. Your doctor is dressed, while you are clad in an unstylish hospital gown or, worse, trying to cover yourself with a large sheet of paper. Your doctor orders the tests; you are the one poked and prodded. Your doctor earns money by caring for you; you pay to be seen. Most important, if things don't go well with your treatments, you are the one who suffers most.

Many valuable relationships are unequal, and they work well *because* they are unequal. Generals are effective leaders when they have power over corporals. Parents can be effective role models and boundary setters *because* they are not on equal footing with their kids. As a patient, understanding how the doctor-patient relationship is unequal will help you use it to your advantage. Your doctors know more about the medical aspects of your illness than you, which helps you! Even for those of you who have become quite expert in your disease, knowing more than your doctors about many aspects of your illness, your doctors still offer you a unique advantage that can help you: They can be objective about your care in a way that you can't. As long as they know enough about you and your medical condition, their objectivity is essential when making certain assessments and decisions.

Being an effective patient means being your own best advocate in everything you do. This sounds fairly simple and straightforward. It's not. Human nature, on the part of both patients and health-care workers, can interfere with healing. Emotions can get in the way of good care. Patients' fear, anger, disappointment, anxiety, embarrassment, resentment, and despair can sabotage taking the necessary steps for healing. Bad experiences with previous doctors lead patients to be skeptical of new doctors who deserve their trust. Doctors who have had trouble with past patients who took a certain approach to healing may sound annoyed to new patients taking similar approaches. Patients who are afraid of appearing stupid may keep their questions to themselves. Doctors who don't like dealing with patients' lists of questions may miss opportunities to help. You and your physicians come into every doctor-patient interaction with a history. Use what you've learned from past experience to make your current relationships work well. If necessary, get help developing healing relationships with the members of your health-care team.

Are you getting the most out of your physicians (generalists, specialists), nurses, physician assistants, allied health-care workers, clergy, family, friends, and other support people?

Communicate! Communicate! Communicate!

You can't expect the members of your health-care team to respond in a helpful or timely fashion when they don't know what you're thinking or feeling.

Tips for Preventing or Overcoming Communication Problems

- Be clear in your own mind about what you hope for, need, expect, and want.
- Create a list that includes important information such as your medications, a complete description of any new symptom (e.g., when the symptom began, what makes it worse), and your questions and concerns. Using a written list decreases your chance of getting sidetracked, running out of time, or forgetting to mention something important during your visit.
- Consider going over your list with a friend or family member before your appointment to ensure you are making sense and including everything that might be important. Consider bringing a close family member or friend to your doctor visits to support or supplement the information you provide.
- Respect your doctor's limitations of time, energy, and patience. Find out what your doctors' needs are regarding calls and visits. Work together to find mutually acceptable times and ways to communicate.
- Establish and nurture an alliance with your doctors so that you can work together toward a shared goal: improving your welfare.

When awkwardness, fear, sadness, or other emotions make it hard for you to talk about a particular topic with your doctor or nurse, try prefacing the information with something like "I feel embarrassed about this, but . . ." or "I'm not sure if this is important or not, but . . ." or "I don't want you to be upset (or disappointed, or frustrated) with me, but . . ." or "It's hard for me to talk about this . . ."

Communication is a two-way process. If you are using a map that you don't know how to read, you may end up in the wrong place. Similarly, if you misunderstand your doctor's directions and advice, your evaluation may not go smoothly and your treatment might not be as safe or effective. Unnecessary suffering can occur if you take the wrong dose of the right pills or you eat foods that are contraindicated. As a Healthy Survivor, make sure you understand completely what your doctors, nurses, or allied health professionals expect you to do before, during, and after each of your visits or treatments.

Tips for Helping You Use Professional Advice

- Bring someone (or a tape recorder) with you to medical visits.
- Write down the findings or conclusions from each call or visit and keep them in a notebook.
- Tell them when you need further explanation and arrange a time to clarify what was said.
- Repeat back your understanding of the directions.

This is *your* healing journey. From the time of diagnosis on, you have many choices about your healing. You choose who is involved in your treatment and recovery and what steps you will take to enhance your recovery. The only way to be an effective patient—finding the best therapies and healers and making wise decisions—is through knowledge, the topic of the next chapter.

What steps can you take to maximize communication with your health-care team? What steps are you taking to ensure that you understand your directions?

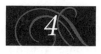

The Role of Knowledge

I *awaken and within seconds remember where I am and why I am here. Instead of jumping out of my nice, warm bed to eat breakfast and read the paper as I usually do before waking my children and getting ready for work, I'm lying in a hospital bed. I'm not going to work today. Right now, I have no idea when I'll be able to return to work, if at all. All I know is that yesterday my colleague (and now, my oncologist) told me that I have small-cell follicular lymphoma. I'm a general internist, not a cancer specialist. The implications of this diagnosis are unclear to me.*

Everything feels wrong: I can't take care of my children or my patients. The idea that this illness might scar my children emotionally, especially if I die, terrifies me more than anything else. On a practical level, I've got an IV line in my arm, surgical bandages on my groin, and thromboguards that feel like suffocating balloons wrapped around my calves. I can't eat or get up by myself. I'm scared of what's happening inside me, afraid of my own body. I'm worried about what I might have to suffer in order to get well, wondering if I can even get well. I feel as if the world stopped and I got off.

Where and how do I begin?

This is the problem: Life as you know it—what I call your "old normal" —collapses in the setting of illness. Medical concerns now demand your attention. Decisions have to be made, possibly the most important ones you've ever made. Routines are disrupted. Roles and relationships change. Your plans for the future dissolve in uncertainty. How can you begin to deal with your diagnosis? What do you have to do to get your life back, both literally and figuratively?

For me, the answers began with knowledge. Obtaining sound knowledge has been essential for me in getting the best medical care and living as fully as possible within the limits of my illness. From the moment of my diagnosis on, obtaining knowledge has been my first step toward Healthy Survivorship. But, wait! While patient advocates proclaim "Knowledge is power" and that knowledge is good, many patients do not use knowledge to their advantage. Why? Because obtaining knowledge is fraught with problems. Knowing certain facts and possibilities can turn your world upside down. To be told you need open-heart surgery is

What specific pieces of information can help you most are unique to you.

frightening and disorienting. Realizing the strain your illness is placing on family members is distressing. To know you could die from your disease—or you are dying—can make your life even more painful. As both a physician and a patient, I am committed to the belief that knowledge is good when you are dealing with illness. But I also believe that what pieces of information constitute an optimal fund of knowledge is unique to each patient.

For instance, some of you need to learn a lot of medical information and some of you need very little, depending upon your medical situation and depending on your personality and style. If you are someone who cannot feel comfortable and confident in your medical care unless you are playing a major role in all the treatment decisions, you need to learn a lot about the medicine of your illness and treatment options, and how to make wise medical decisions. And if it just so happens that you are spooked by statistics, you also need to learn new ways of thinking about statistics so that you can use them when weighing your choices. If this sounds like you, chapters 5 and 6 will be of interest to you.

Conversely, if you don't want to make medical decisions or you absolutely can't deal with statistics without becoming distressed, you still can become a Healthy Survivor. Instead of learning the ins and outs of your treatment options, you can focus your attention on finding a highly competent physician who is willing and able to make all your medical decisions. You can avoid all mention of statistics and, instead, talk about your treatment options in terms of your overall goals. To suggest that you *must* be intimately involved in the medical decisions or that you must learn to talk about statistics isn't fair, and it would only hurt you. Depending on your needs and desires, you can skim or skip the parts of chapters 5 and 6 that aren't helping you. And that is fine. Because one style of survivorship is not better than another, as long as you are getting good care.

Here lies the rub: No matter the makeup of your personality, you have to learn *enough* to get good care. In my opinion, if you are suffering unnecessarily because you are not informed about good options for resolving your problem, be it a medical or a nonmedical one, you need more knowledge. If you don't know the warning signs and symptoms of complications, you can't take good care of yourself between office visits. This chapter and the two that follow assume that you don't want to suffer when suffering is avoidable and you want to survive, if survival with an acceptable quality of life is a reasonable possibility. If you can't focus on gaining this knowledge, appoint a family member or friend to do the reading for you and rely on her or him to discuss medical matters with you.

To become a Healthy Survivor, you have to determine how much knowledge works best for you, which means you have to know yourself and be true to yourself. Since I believe you need to learn a minimum, throughout the next three chapters I'll point out when I consider information to be essential to Healthy Survivorship. Beyond that, the information and advice are geared to those of you who need or want to be very involved and proactive. Learn as much or as little as is necessary to both get good care and live as fully as possible.

In this chapter, I discuss many of the ways that knowledge can help you, physically and emotionally. I outline some problems associated with knowledge and offer ways to deal with them. My goal is to help you see knowledge not as a threat but as an opportunity, so that you can use knowledge to your advantage.

A Patient's View of Knowledge

When I had my medical practice, Sir Francis Peabody's adage about "curing as often as possible and comforting always" guided my everyday work. To this end, I spent an enormous amount of time and energy educating my patients. Explaining what was going on in terms my patients understood calmed them before I'd done anything tangible for them. Outlining and discussing the options for evaluating and treating their problems seemed to help them find hope and strength, and adjust to the changes. This education helped them accept the outcome, even when things didn't go well despite everyone's best efforts. Not only were patients and I a more effective team when they were knowledgeable, I also found it easier and more fun to care for them. It made perfect sense to me when I learned that the word *doctor* was derived from the Latin *docere*—to teach—because every day I saw how providing sound information helped heal patients.

When I became a patient, I experienced in a whole new way the almost magical healing power of knowledge. During the most awful times, sound knowledge about what to expect calmed my fears more than the loving reassurances of friends and family. Practical advice, even when I didn't like the recommendation, helped me feel less alone and inspired me to carry on. Feeling that I'd made informed decisions helped me find acceptance, no matter what was happening medically. The doctrine that I'd trusted as a physician I now knew to be true as a patient: Knowledge can help you deal with what is happening in healthy ways. Knowledge helps you to get the most out of your treatments and your relationships with your physicians and nurses. Knowledge helps you to take good care of yourself between office visits. It helps you relate to family and friends, too, and manage the emotional and financial burdens as painlessly as possible. Comfort and hope arise from understanding what is happening to you and being able to communicate well with those who can help. Most important of all, empowerment stems from knowing the various ways you can affect what is happening.

> From the time of diagnosis on, knowledge can help you let go of worry and focus on living.

How well do you feel that you understand what is happening to you physically? Emotionally? How well do you know what to expect in the future? How well prepared do you feel for dealing with upcoming challenges?

Knowing When You Are a Patient

You wear many different hats—worker, friend, child, sibling, parent, committee member, and neighbor, to name just a few. Which hats you might be wearing at any instant depends upon your situation at the moment. Whatever your medical challenge, while you are being evaluated or treated one of the hats you are wearing is that of patient. You can feel perfectly healthy and be working eighty hours a week as a corporate executive, but if you have a medical problem you are also a patient.

If my cancer diagnosis gave me no choice about becoming a patient, I did have a choice about what kind of patient I became. I've tried to be an effective patient, namely one who gets good care. Sir William Osler's warning rings in my head: "A physician who treats himself has a fool for a patient." The words of this renowned nineteenth-century physician make clear one of the essential characteristics of a healing physician-patient relationship: Obtaining knowledge is not intended as a way for patients to take over their own care and free themselves of dependency on the expertise and goodwill of others. Rather, effective patients obtain knowledge for three reasons:

1. to help their doctors direct their care;
2. to care for themselves as much as is possible and wise; and
3. to obtain support, medical and otherwise, when needed.

As a Healthy Survivor, you don't need to know everything about your illness; you need to know *enough*. Some patients become experts on their conditions, and that works well for them. But it might be better for you to learn the minimum needed to be an effective patient and get good care. When I started my first round of chemotherapy, I didn't know much beyond the few facts remembered from my residency days about the drugs flowing into my narrow veins. As a general internist, I'd never prescribed or administered chemotherapy. Much to the surprise of some, I didn't pore over textbooks of pharmacology and try to become an expert in my treatment regimen. I felt that my energies were better used elsewhere—adjusting to the changes and helping my children. I did learn what I needed to know about the drugs to be an effective patient, and then I trusted my oncologist to know what he needed to know to take good care of me. Healthy Survivors learn enough to be able to trust their physicians and feel secure in the treatments their doctors prescribe.

Implicit in the notion of being an effective patient is your willingness and ability to trust others to care for you. The best chest surgeon in the world can't perform a coronary bypass on himself. A grief counselor leans on others after a personal loss. All patients have times of needing to depend on others. The key is knowing whom to trust and how to trust.

How do you use knowledge to help your physicians care for you? How do you decide who is worthy of your trust? What decisions are you facing?

Basic Knowledge Needed

Illness introduces a host of big and little choices in all spheres of your life. As a Healthy Survivor, you want to make the best decisions at every phase of your survivorship. Which doctors and clinics will you use? Which treatments will you take? How do you want to relate to your health-care team? How are you going to divide up your energy, especially if it is limited? What will you do about your obligations at home, work, or school? How are your expectations and goals for the future going to change, if at all? How will you manage your finances now that you have the added burden of medical expenses and lost income? How are your roles in life

and your relationships with others going to change in the short run? In
the long run? How much and what kind of support are you willing to
accept? What are you going to tell your children about your situation?
How hopeful are you going to be? Decisions, decisions, decisions. These
are just a few of the many decisions Healthy Survivors make as they deal
with medical challenges. Knowledge opens your eyes to good options and
then helps you weigh one against another.

Obtain Knowledge About

Medical Issues
>your disease or injury, in general
>your specific medical condition
>your treatment options
>your particular treatments

Nonmedical Issues: the effects of your illness on your
>emotional state
>psychological state
>social circumstances
>spirituality
>finances

Decision Making
>how to make wise decisions in the context of your specific illness

Support
>support for yourself and family during illness

In order to make wise decisions that affect your survivorship positively, what, exactly, do you need to know? It depends. At the very least,
you need to learn the basics about your disease, your current medical
condition, and your treatments. It also helps you to understand how your
life has changed and, just as important, how it hasn't. You need some
understanding of the effect of your illness on the social, intellectual,
emotional, spiritual, and financial aspects of your life. Since you will be

making decisions that affect your situation, it is essential that you know how to make wise decisions. And you need to understand the role of support in your survivorship and how to obtain it.

The need for knowledge doesn't stop after you've completed the diagnosis and evaluation phases and started on a course of treatment. My ongoing education about my survivorship has enabled me to ride the ups, downs, and straightaways of long-term survivorship, be it the discomforts of treatment, the emotional high of a new remission, the transition of recovery, the strain of routine checkups, and the distress of cancer recurrences and aftereffects. From the time of the diagnosis on, Healthy Survivors obtain knowledge.

> You don't need to know everything; you need to know enough.

Choice

For years, I prescribed treatments for my patients. Underlying the ritual of writing prescriptions in front of my patients was our shared belief that we could affect what was happening now and might happen in the future, and that we could increase the chances of a good outcome by making wise choices. Obviously you can't change what's happening to your body if you have no choice about it. But you also won't take steps to change what's happening if *you think* that you can't do anything about it. Knowledge helps you know when you have options and what those options are. Knowledge enables you to find and pursue the best options for you.

Have you ever bought something, thinking that the particular item you purchased was the only one you could get, and then learned that a better model was available, or an equally good but less expensive model? One day, I needed a single poster board but ended up buying a package of ten because I didn't know that the store also sold them singly. Another time, my husband and I went to a lovely restaurant to celebrate our anniversary, and we ordered from the menu. As our waiter set our entrees in front of us, I overheard another waiter telling the patrons at the next table about the "Special of the Day"—a dish I hadn't known was available and would have preferred.

Of course, when dealing with illness, the consequences of not knowing your treatment options can be far more disastrous than making an uneconomical purchase or eating a disappointing meal. You may need to consult more than one doctor to find out about your best options. Sarah sought the opinion of a new neurologist, who prescribed medication that brought her relief from her frequent migraines. She was grateful but also angry that her headaches had been uncontrolled for so long because she had been taking a less effective medication prescribed by the neurologist who'd been following her for years. Mark feels guilty about his divorce. He is now aware that had he taken advantage of available support services, divorce may have been avoided. If you don't ever want to say "I wish I knew *then* what I know *now*," knowledge is the key.

> If you don't ever want to say "I wish I knew then what I know now," knowledge is the key.

Do you feel you have enough information about your treatment? Managing your symptoms, such as nausea or pain? Your physicians? Your support system? Your sense of hope?

Windows of Opportunity

Have you ever seen a bug accidentally fly into a room and the only exit is a window opened just a crack? I remember as a child watching with fascination a bee in my basement, buzzing around the window, trying to get back outside. Smack. Bump. The bee kept smashing into the clear glass. He hit the center of the glass, the top, and then both sides, over and over. Finally, bruised and tired, he swooped low and slipped out the opening at the bottom of the window. If only he had known ahead of time how to get out.

The first few weeks after my diagnosis, the doctor visits, treatment decisions, uncertainty, and discomforts made me feel trapped in my situation. I didn't want to be like that bee, randomly bumping my way to freedom. Knowledge was my safest and fastest way out. Maybe you've heard the phrase "When a door closes, a window opens . . . it's those long dark hallways that are tough." Knowledge is like a light in a long dark hallway, revealing the way to and through open windows of opportunity. You may be stopped in your tracks by fear of your disease or confusion over how to balance the demands of your job and the demands of your treatments. It is knowledge that shows you healthy ways to deal with the challenges and to move beyond crippling indecision.

The captain of an ocean liner was notorious for his belligerent stubbornness. One dark night, while cruising along at a fast clip, the ship received a message in code from a blinking light twenty knots ahead, "This is Freedom Day. You are headed straight for us. Please change direction." The captain, upon receiving this message, ordered his communications officer to send this message, "I am staying on course. *You* change *your* direction!" Within moments, the captain's ship received another signal: "This is Freedom Day. I'm not moving." The captain bristled, unwilling to have someone else tell him what to do. As the distance between Freedom Day and the ship narrowed dangerously, he sent one last warning: "I am NOT changing direction." Freedom Day responded, "I'm not changing direction, either. I'm a lighthouse."

This parable illustrates the value of recognizing when your chosen path is headed toward disaster. Some treatments can tempt you with false visions of good results but, in reality, only keep you from useful treatments. Knowledge of unrealistic goals helps you maintain your momentum toward healing. Don't be like James, a patient who consulted doctor after doctor, delaying needed treatment because none of the doctors would guarantee him a cure, or like Frances, who declined the one treatment that might have cured her because she insisted on taking a nonsurgical approach. Knowledge helps you avoid unrealistic goals about the non-medical challenges, too. When you learn that a normal and healthy reaction to medical setbacks includes temporary feelings of fear and hopelessness, you won't expect yourself and those around you to remain calm and unflinchingly optimistic in the face of bad news about your condition. By keeping you as safe as possible, and by keeping your energies channeled toward productive pursuits, knowledge can help you to live as fully as possible while getting good care. Knowledge about options and limits is essential to Healthy Survivorship.

How often do you feel trapped? How often do you bump up against limits? Are you tempted by easy solutions to difficult problems? Are you pursuing any goals that are unrealistic?

Knowledge about Limits

In survivorship, knowing about limits is crucial. When thinking about my limits, I often picture a balloon. Let me explain. I'm someone who likes to do a lot, so my personal goal, metaphorically speaking, is to blow up my balloon as big as I can. Knowing when my balloon is nearing its maximum size helps me. And it helps to know ahead of time approximately how big my balloon can get. If I don't have any sense of my limits, I might watch other people's balloons grow bigger than mine, and keep blowing and blowing until . . . POP! . . . my balloon explodes in my face. When you don't know your limits, things can go badly. If you lift too much after surgery, you might tear your incision. If you push yourself too hard when you are overtired, you might fall asleep at the steering wheel of your car. All human beings have limits. During and after treatment, your limits may be greater, at least for a while. In most cases, it helps you to learn about your limits.

Those caring for you have limits, too. Spouses, lovers, parents, friends, and even professional health-care workers can't do everything, be everywhere, and understand everything all the time. They are just people. They can take only so much physical and emotional stress. If you don't recognize or respect the limits of those who care for and about you, gentleness and generosity may give way to hurtful words or actions that compromise your relationships. Even faith can have limits that are exposed by your illness. A strong belief in a higher power can include times of doubting and questioning when things are going badly, especially when your thinking may be affected by drugs, pain, or fatigue. If you expect your faith to be unwavering under all circumstances, you may abandon what could have been a tremendous source of comfort and strength.

Knowing your limits is not enough. You need to respect them. Maybe you are having trouble accepting that you are sick or don't want to ask others for help. You might be someone who subscribes to the macho school of self-healing, believing that the harder you push yourself the faster you'll get better. Or, following your doctors' and nurses' instructions may feel like you've lost total control of your life, especially if you are being advised to change the way you do tasks as mundane as brushing your teeth. If this sounds like you, remember that respecting your limits is one way to regain some control over your life. Respecting your limits can free you of the burden of many *preventable* problems. It's fine to feel as if you have no limits as long as you take care of yourself. It's not okay to act as if you have no limits when doing so hurts you, your loved ones, or those who are depending on you.

Unless you're ready for it, you may get confused and discouraged by going three steps forward, one step backward, two steps forward, one step backward, and so on. As you receive and recover from treatment, your stamina, patience, appetite, ability to concentrate, and hopefulness may fluctuate from week to week, even day to day or hour to hour.

> Respecting your limits is one way to regain some control over your life.

Returning to the balloon metaphor may help. As you move from the crisis of your diagnosis through your treatments to recovery, the size of your balloon is getting bigger and smaller, bigger and smaller, again and again. Once you enter the recovery stage, if everything goes smoothly, each subsequent balloon should be a little bigger. In other words, you'll be able to handle more and more as time passes. When complications or setbacks occur, your current balloon will be replaced with a smaller one, possibly forever. Obtaining knowledge about limits will help you know when your balloon has been replaced with a smaller one so you don't blow too hard and pop it.

The other problem is *under*estimating your limits. It would be a shame if you had a big balloon with a fabulously intricate design but never blew it up all the way because you were afraid to pop it. You couldn't appreciate the full effect of the design and color. Similarly, in addition to knowing what you can't do and shouldn't try to do, it helps to know what you *can* do. A seeming paradox, knowing your limits can free you by giving you the confidence to do more, to help you not give up too early or too much. One hairdresser who suffers from treatment-related fatigue arranged to use a chair with a high seat and legs on casters that roll with little effort. So instead of being bored and depressed at home with little social contact and no income, she is sitting comfortably while cutting her clients' hair. Knowing how to expand to reach her full limits, she enjoys her work and income. Another survivor is afraid to ask his pregnant sister for support. A counselor encourages him to talk openly with her, and he finds out that she had been feeling helpless and now is grateful for the opportunity to be involved. Knowing the nature of your limits can help free you to live most fully.

> Knowing your limits frees you to do more and not give up too early or too much.

How well do you know your limits? How well do you respect your limits? How well do you know others' limits? Who can help you determine how your limits are changing from day to day, week to week?

Risk versus Benefit

Everything in life carries risks and benefits. When you love someone, you believe that it is better to have loved and lost than never to have loved at all. When you lend your valuables to a friend, you feel that sharing is more important than the possibility of not getting your valuables back in the same condition, if at all. Every decision you make reflects not only your assessment of what you'll get but also what it might cost you if you go that route. To make wise decisions and move forward, you need to know the risks and benefits of each of your choices, medical and otherwise, and you need to be able to weigh them fairly.

When your physicians recommend a treatment, they've already made a calculation that the potential benefits to you outweigh the risks. When your physician prescribes pain medication, the possibility of side effects or complications such as an allergic reaction and the price of the drugs are weighed against the expected benefits. If you want to help your physician tailor medical treatments to your personal needs and preferences, you must understand the risks and benefits of your treatment options.

Regarding nonmedical challenges of survivorship, such as problems in your relationships with your friends and family, obtaining knowledge is the best way to assess the risks and benefits of the various ways to approach the problems. Look at Sherry, a middle-aged woman whose marriage was rocky before she was diagnosed with cancer. By learning about the effects of family illness on unstable marriages, she gained a sense of the advantages and disadvantages of sticking it out with her husband through treatment versus going through a divorce now. Cynthia was a dedicated mom who was inclined to keep her unexpected diagnosis of diabetes a secret from her children because she had no idea how to break the news. Besides, she wanted to protect them from worrying. By learning about the effects of family illness on youngsters, she understood the benefits of open communication, and she acquired the skills and confidence needed to tell each of her children about her illness in life-enhancing ways.

Knowledge about risks and benefits can help you find hope. Robert is in despair, dealing with chronic heart failure. A social worker teaches him about the risks and benefits of repression and denial, and about the various types of hope. He learns how to nourish genuine hope in a bleak situation, and he is helped by his newfound ability to feel hope with acceptance. Janice, after her heart muscle was damaged beyond repair by a viral illness, finds hope for the first time after learning about the risks and benefits of heart transplant, an option that terrified her before she learned more about it.

*How well do you know the risks and benefits of each approach
to the problems you are facing?*

Obstacles to Obtaining Knowledge

We are living in the Information Age, yet many patients are stumped by obstacles to obtaining sound knowledge about their illness. Mable lived on a farm in rural Texas and didn't have easy access to a computer or cancer-support services. In contrast, Leslie lived in Dallas and could find information easily enough but found everything too technical and hard to understand. Maybe you have a rare illness or you have other medical conditions that complicate matters so that little information exists that applies to you and few professionals have experience with your situation. Accurate, useful information too easily blurs with the well-intended but misinformed advice of friends and family. The effects of pain, fatigue, and medications take a toll when trying to concentrate and learn new information. And misconceptions keep patients from learning about healthy ways to deal with their pain or fatigue, or marital and financial stress. It may never cross your mind that services exist not only to help you minimize your pain and fatigue but also to counsel you through your family problems or assist with your medical bills. So you don't find out about these useful services, and you suffer the consequences.

My professional life revolved around obtaining and using medical information. Yet after my diagnosis, when treatment was needed urgently because I had terrible pain from a tumor pressing on a major nerve, I was too sick and shocked to participate in the decision making in any meaningful way. My disorientation and confusion didn't resolve upon being discharged from the hospital, either. I didn't even realize how poorly I was functioning until almost a year later when I rearranged my bedroom furniture as a symbolic act to help me put my cancer experience behind me. Moving my bed, I uncovered a short stack of informational patient handouts on chemotherapy on the dusty carpet. The material was terrific, so I brought the pamphlets to my chemo nurse, Brenda, expecting her to thank me. She looked at me as if I were joking around. Realizing that I was serious, she said, "Wendy, I gave these pamphlets to you at your first chemotherapy session." I still don't remember getting them.

My husband—the philosophy-loving professor of political economy—stopped by the local medical-school library on his way home from the hospital on the day of my original diagnosis. But it was weeks before I could bring myself to open one of my own medical textbooks. When I finally mustered the nerve to read the section on my type of lymphoma, the opening statement immobilized me for days: "This cancer invariably recurs . . . with shorter and shorter remissions . . . and leads to death."

The textbook with the death sentence may have contained the most up-to-date information that could help me evaluate and care for my patients. But reading the textbook *as a patient* did not help me until I learned a new way to read this sort of information. Concepts I knew as a physician—prognosis, hope, trust—I had to learn all over again as a patient. Over the years, the course of my illness did not match the textbook's predictions. The textbooks have since been rewritten, and I've learned to use technical medical information in ways that help me as a patient.

Throughout survivorship, one of the greatest obstacles to obtaining sound knowledge for many patients is emotions. Despite loads of solid information being thrown at patients, their emotions—their shock, fear, anxiety, confusion, anger, mistrust, and sadness—can make it difficult for them to hear what others are saying at times. Feelings of hopelessness can keep patients from making the effort to pursue second opinions. Anger at family members can keep patients from listening to useful advice.

Not only can emotions be obstacles to obtaining knowledge in the first place, but emotions can also become obstacles after you begin to obtain knowledge. You might start off feeling calm and confident, but as you learn about your medical condition, social situation, or financial state, you may begin to feel afraid, discouraged, angry, guilty, disappointed, helpless, or confused. Your emotions don't have to sabotage Healthy Survivorship. Chapter 7 discusses using your emotions in ways that help you to get good care and to live fully.

Let me take a moment here to mention briefly one emotion that can make your illness like the elephant in the living room no one acknowledges: fear. Fear of learning upsetting facts and fear of saying or doing the wrong things can keep you from finding out what you need to know to prevent and overcome problems. Years ago, when I was talking with a friend one night about the fear that arises when new symptoms develop, our conversation was getting bogged down. Always one to try a little comedy, I joked, "I know a way to tame my anxiety: get a frontal lobotomy! Then I'd know what my symptom might mean, but I wouldn't care!" My silliness worked, bringing relief as we laughed about something very painful. The punch line pointed to the crux of the issue: Physical symptoms and tensions in relationships trigger fear, and this fear is uncomfortable. As will be discussed in chapter 7, fear is not all bad. Fear becomes a problem only when it keeps you from obtaining knowledge or doing what you need to do to help your situation.

A frontal lobotomy or mind-numbing drugs may be tempting when distressed, but they are terrible ways to deal with fear. In most cases, the best way to tame fears is to face them, often with the guidance and support of others. Ignorance is not bliss when you are a patient. Healthy Survivors learn how to overcome the obstacles to obtaining sound knowledge.

What obstacles are keeping you from obtaining sound knowledge? What specific fears are keeping you from obtaining knowledge? How can you get past these fears to find the knowledge you need now?

Antianxiety Drugs

I must digress for a moment. Although I strongly discourage you from self-medicating with drugs or alcohol or using any unsafe behavior in an attempt to escape the stress of your medical situation, physician-prescribed antianxiety medications may be an important element in your getting good care. Emotional distress can make it difficult—sometimes, too difficult—for you to process the information provided by your health-care team. Anxiety can make it hard to do what you need to do to get better, such as undergo tests and receive treatment, or even eat and sleep. Safe and effective antianxiety medication prescribed by your physician can make it possible for you to hear and understand important information and to do the right thing when you couldn't otherwise. As you adjust to your diagnosis and learn what you can do about what's happening, or as you begin to treat your illness, your anxiety level will likely diminish and you won't need medication anymore. If your illness is persistent, you may need long-term medication to function as normally as possible under the extraordinary circumstances.

Regrettably, myth and stigma surround the use of antianxiety drugs. People deny themselves the benefit of medications because they fear becoming addicted or overmedicated. Recent concerns about the link between the use of certain antidepressants and the risk of suicide make people wary of any mood-altering medication. For patients who are feeling that their world is out of control already, the idea of taking pills for their nervousness seems paramount to letting go of one of the last areas of their lives over which they have control. Or they see taking medication as evidence that they are weak, or that they've gone crazy. In fact, people who need antianxiety medication in a crisis don't become addicted or overmedicated, assuming that the drugs are prescribed by a qualified physician. Taking needed medications indicates wisdom and strength in challenging circumstances and gives you back a sense of control by helping you think and act more like your usual self. The goal is to get information that will help you. If you need a little pharmacological help from your doctors in order to get second opinions or proceed with certain tests, go for it!

A Lifesaving Key

Here's a parable that illustrates different ways to deal with the emotional discomfort of acquiring useful information. Sam, Saul, Stephen, and Solomon are each locked in separate soundproof rooms with no food or water. The only way out is with a key that is kept in a box that gives off an electric shock when touched.

Sam tries to retrieve the key from the box. When shocked, he stops all efforts to escape and curls up in a corner, destined to die of starvation unless a miracle occurs.

Saul, too, gets shocked when he tries to get the key. Instead of giving up, though, Saul looks around and uses his pocketknife to cut the electric cable to the box. Now it's possible for him to slip his hand into the box, grab the key, and unlock the door to safety.

Stephen, like Saul, looks for a way to avoid a shock but can't find a pocketknife or other tool to disable the current. Thinking creatively, he makes a buffer by wrapping a piece of his shirt around his fingers. Now he is somewhat insulated, and he grabs the key without getting shocked too badly.

Last, poor Solomon has no tools or clothing in the room. Knowing that time is running out and that unlocking the door is his only chance of survival, he takes a deep breath and grabs the key. He cries out as the electric current burns his fingers. Yet using the key to unlock the door, Solomon survives. With time, his wounds heal.

Some information is vital to getting good care, such as knowing the signs and symptoms of problems that need medical attention. When learning essential information makes you upset or anxious, try to find a way to minimize your discomfort without compromising the usefulness of the facts. One way is to make the painful part less so, like Saul or Stephen, such as by distracting or detaching yourself from the upsetting aspects. For example, if you learn about a potential complication, you can focus on the likelihood that it will never develop or that it is treatable. When you simply can't find any way to soften the distress, don't give up. Take a deep breath, focus on the useful information that can help you, and bear the pain. Take comfort and strength in knowing that your pain is temporary, like that of Solomon's burns. Whatever you do, don't be like Sam, who shuts down at the first hint of pain. Avoiding acute pain may consign you to suffer chronic pain or loss down the line. It's amazing what you can endure for a short while.

Are you most like Sam, Saul, Stephen, or Solomon?

Choosing Not to Know

What if you really don't want to know? What if you don't want to face facts that might help you? What if you don't want to know the truth about your medical situation? I've known (and you've probably known) people who don't ever want to know the risk of choices they are making, such as the risks associated with continued smoking. Some patients don't want to know their prognosis, especially if the predictions are pessimistic. They don't want to hear, ever, that their disease or treatment may cause them to suffer. Some patients make it clear that they'd prefer lies over learning that they are dying. Can these people be Healthy Survivors, too? Isn't it presumptuous of me to say that knowing is better than not knowing? Isn't this a question of personal choice? Won't some people's lives be better—happier—if they don't really understand the gravity of their situations or their choices?

Only you can know how much knowledge will help you become a Healthy Survivor. If learning certain pieces of information overwhelms your ability to do or enjoy anything, having it forced down your throat is cruel. Knowledge that immobilizes you is not useful information, no matter how "essential" it may seem. You need to explore your primary goals (comfort? living longer?), and you need to know yourself. These are philosophical issues that are complex and highly personal. From the standpoint of Healthy Survivorship, you have to know a minimum to get good care. Ironically, choosing not to know certain things may be essential to your living fully.

I have thought long and hard about if I would want to know if I had a high risk of developing some major medical disaster ten years hence. Would I want to know if I were dying? My answer has been "Yes, it is better for me to know" because this knowledge helps me make good decisions. Knowing the truth about my situation enables me to discuss my needs and my treatment options with the members of my health-care team, thus helping them help me. Being informed about the effect of my illness on my family makes it possible for me to respond in ways that help us work together to get through the hard times. And, when I'm dying— be it a year from now or forty years from now—I believe that facing the truth will help me make the most of whatever time I have left.

The essential question for me is not "Should I learn the truth about the bad stuff?" but "What should I do with the information that is upsetting me?" Learning the truth may make me unhappy at first, but the truth frees me to make wise choices and move on. In many cases, the harsh truth motivates me to do things that, otherwise, I'd find hard to do. My goal in dealing with my illness has been to move beyond it and live as meaningful and joyful a life as I can within the limits of my illness, in what time I have. The only way that I, Wendy, can find true happiness is if I am living in a world where I know the truth about what is happening to me, to the degree that anyone can know the truth. By learning the truth about my condition and understanding its ripple effect on all aspects of my life, I can decide what to do about it. But, that is me. What about you?

How much do you want to know?

Finding Balance

What if, instead of being like those who try to ignore new symptoms and avoid learning about the effects of their illness on their life, you start monitoring every little ache or pain and want to know as much as possible about each and every aspect of survivorship. Does the suggestion to obtain knowledge mean you are supposed to call your doctor every time you notice a change or feel different in some way? Are you supposed to surf the Internet or go to the library and research every new medication that is prescribed for you? Are you supposed to analyze every tense interchange with friends and loved ones? No, of course not. Your whole life does not have to revolve around your illness just because you have an illness.

Healthy Survivors find a balance that works best for them. Find a balance of times when it is best if you find out more about your situation and when it is best to let go and trust what the members of your health-care team are doing. When you aren't sure if you are being too blasé or too vigilant about a symptom or problem, ask the appropriate members of your health-care team, "Should I be worried about this?"

Knowing a lot of facts may give you some sense of control, and researching new treatments may give you a sense of hope, but you need to ask yourself if these efforts to obtain more knowledge are helping you get better care and live more fully. I've seen patients get completely wrapped up in researching and talking about their disease. Instead of using knowledge to create an alliance with their physicians, they use it as ammunition in what becomes an adversarial relationship with the people who can help them. Instead of using knowledge to make their lives better, their obsessive search for information and answers makes them prisoners to their disease, even when they are doing well medically!

Healthy Survivors develop a sense of when enough is enough. They know when questions or problems don't have a definitive answer, or a "best" or "good" answer. And, some questions don't have any answers. For example, back in 1993 I could have researched forever and yet never experienced a moment of "Eureka! I found the ultimate right answer for treating this cancer recurrence." Instead, the best I could do was to find some realistic treatment options, suboptimal as they were, and make an educated decision with my physicians about which one seemed the best for me. Obtaining knowledge is a means to an end, not an end in itself. When the best answer is no answer, or a less than optimal one, recognize that you know enough to make the best decisions you can regarding your health and your life, and move on.

How much is enough is unique to each individual. Figuring out when enough is enough reminds me of the dilemma of looking for a lost valuable, such as an heirloom wedding band. If you were fairly sure that you lost it in a particular room but you weren't positive, how long would you look? How would you decide when to stop looking? When dealing with uncertainty, you have to make a judgment call about when to accept the answers you have, even if they are unsatisfactory. If the ring *is* in the room somewhere and you give up the search too soon, you'll never find it. If the ring *is not* in the room, time and energy you spend looking there is wasted because you'll never find what you are looking for. In a similar way, if you don't get enough information, you may sacrifice opportunities to improve your situation. Conversely, if you don't know when to stop, your efforts to obtain knowledge can become counterproductive to your well-being and to finding happiness. Learn to judge when you have enough information to be an effective patient and live fully. Maybe the answer will become clear if you answer another question: "What do I need to know to get good care, feel better, and live my life fully?" For me, I feel I have enough knowledge when I understand what is going on, know what to do to increase my chances of doing well, and have answers with which I can live.

How much information do you need to be a Healthy Survivor? Why are you continuing to obtain knowledge? When will you feel that you have enough information?

Resources for Obtaining Sound Knowledge

How can you overcome the obstacles to obtaining sound knowledge? How can you develop this sense of balance and learn to respond appropriately to warning signs and symptoms? Nowadays, you don't have to fight your way through the ups and downs of survivorship all by yourself. The first and most important step is developing working alliances with your doctors and nurses and the rest of your health-care team. Your physicians and nurses are a key source of medical information, especially as regards your self-monitoring and the reporting of physical signs or symptoms. They also can refer you to allied health professionals who can guide and support you through nonmedical challenges that arise. Over time, and with experience, you'll become adept at knowing what to look for, how to care for yourself between office visits, and how to get proper attention. You'll also know when and how to move on.

The experience of veteran survivors and the expertise of professionals can provide a map, warning you of potential problems and offering tips for preventing and overcoming them. Over the months following completion of my first course of chemotherapy, I learned of resources that would have been helpful had I known about them earlier. It was only be-cause I'd become active in survivorship with my writing and advocacy work that I found out about many of them at all. I am embarrassed by how little I knew before my diagnosis about the informational and supportive services available outside my hospital. I take little comfort in the realization that my deficiency was common among conventionally trained physicians and, I suspect, is still the norm.

In order to satisfy your personal needs for information and encourage optimal relationships with your physicians and nurses, it often helps to get additional information from other resources. For almost all major diseases, national and local organizations and Web sites run by professionals or institutions can provide reliable, accurate information about your specific disease, and can refer you to additional good information and support resources.

Do you know when to call your physicians and nurses about a problem? Do you ask them for referrals for nonmedical problems? Are you using local and national resources to your best advantage?

As will be discussed fully in chapter 5, not all information available to you is of the same quality. Even well-educated people can find it hard to separate the good from the bad, the safe from the dangerous. A theory or article can sound scientific when, in fact, it is not scientific at all. Pseudoscience can be perilous. Check with your physicians when you obtain information that might affect what you do. Indications that information may be misleading or wrong include: old publication dates, use of anecdotes and testimonials to support claims, credentials that are not recognized by responsible scientists or educators, lack of scientific evidence, and references that are outdated, irrelevant, untraceable, or based on poorly designed research. Healthy Survivors rely on information that is sound.

Knowing When and How to Delegate

To a degree, it is possible for you to become a Healthy Survivor without learning about your illness or treatment options. You could delegate the job to a family member or friend who is willing and able to work with your physicians and to serve as your advocate when weighing treatment options and making decisions. Delegating to others may be necessary at times when you can't or shouldn't obtain knowledge or make decisions. You may be too stressed, physically or emotionally, by your current medical condition to learn about it or make wise decisions. Or, you might be in the midst of another life crisis when suddenly you are faced with serious illness. You might be struggling through a divorce, grieving the sudden death of a loved one, or distressed by the unexpected loss of your job or home. You may want to participate actively in the decision making but, for whatever reason, you are not in a position to obtain or process information. In fact, it may be counterproductive for you to try to do so right now. That's fine as long as someone else can take over this job until you can become involved yourself.

Who can learn for you and advocate for you, when you can't do it yourself? What are the times when you'd do best to delegate the job of obtaining knowledge?

Moving On

Obtaining sound knowledge is the first step in tackling your illness, so you can move on with your life. Once you recognize and overcome the many obstacles to obtaining knowledge, you can use sound information to shape your reality in positive ways. Chapter 5 discusses how to obtain knowledge about your medical condition now that you are ready to find it.

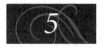

Mastering Medical Knowledge

*T*he woman repeated her friend's question before answering, "You want to know what treatment they give me? Gee, I don't know. I never ask my doctors any questions about my condition or treatment. They tell me where I have to be and when, and I show up."

Why should you obtain medical knowledge? Why not let the experts take over your medical care completely? The answer is simple: You need at least a minimum of medical knowledge to get good care, no matter how active or passive a role you choose to play in the decisions regarding your evaluation and treatment. And, whether you like it or not, in the end you are the one responsible for your health, not your doctors, nurses, or care-givers. This chapter, based on the ideas presented in chapter 4 regarding the role of knowledge in general, focuses on medical knowledge. It discusses overcoming obstacles to obtaining medical information and evaluating the quality of that information. This is not a guide to medical information about your disease but, rather, a method for mastering medical information so that you can use it to your advantage.

What Is Happening?

Serious illness sweeps you into the medical world of unknowns: "What's happening to my body now?" "What is going to happen to me in the future?" "What are they (the doctors, nurses, and technicians) doing?" After the diagnosis is made, patients experience an overwhelming sense of loss of control over their world, especially at first. If you can't speak the language used to discuss your illness, how can you understand what's going on or communicate with those who do, let alone influence your outcome in positive ways? Without medical knowledge, your feeling that your health is out of your control, and the fears and anxieties this loss triggers, are magnified. Having at least a minimum of medical knowledge helps you a tremendous amount.

Thinking about how medical knowledge helps newly diagnosed patients brings to my mind an image: People are standing at the ocean's edge just as a powerful wave reaches the shore. For those who have never been to a beach and who've been told nothing, the wave sweeps them out into the salty seas where they swallow water and flail their arms uselessly. For those who have been instructed briefly on what to expect and do, the first big wave still knocks them off balance, but instead of panicking they rise to the surface, catch their breath, and stay afloat until the next wave comes, and they swim safely to shore. Medical knowledge helps you ride the big and little waves of illness.

I have friends and relatives who prefer to let their health-care team tell them exactly what to do at every step of the way. Maybe you are like them, wanting to focus all your energies on the nonmedical aspects of what is happening such as adjusting emotionally to the changes or strengthening your faith. You may want to learn the least of the medical side as you possibly can to get by. The scientific and technical aspects of your illness may seem too complex and sophisticated, time-consuming, or emotionally upsetting.

> Basic medical knowledge helps you to minimize the pain, debility, and loss due to your illness.

As mentioned in the introduction to chapter 4, how much medical information you need is unique to you. It depends on your medical condition and on you—your needs and desires, your personality and style. But choosing to learn nothing about the medical aspects of your illness is counter to Healthy Survivorship because you may miss opportunities to preserve your health should problems arise between office visits.

When Medical Knowledge Seems Overwhelming

If the medical side of your illness feels like a lot (too much!) to learn, think back to when you learned how to drive a car. At first, you had to concentrate on each and every step before you could get going: Fasten your safety belt, place your foot on the brake, adjust your rear- and side-view mirrors, turn on the ignition, release the parking brake, shift into drive, check the road, check your blind spot, lift your foot off the brake, and gently push down on the accelerator. Within a few days this series of maneuvers became more automatic and, consequently, easier. So, too, when your diagnosis is new it may feel like an overwhelming amount to learn, partly because the situation involves new jargon and a lot of facts and feelings. Just as most people can learn to drive a car, most people can learn the medical information they need to know.

Depending upon the urgency of your need for medical treatment, you may be able to start your education in a fairly relaxed mode or you may need a crash course. It also depends on how much you can handle, physically and emotionally. You may be too sick or distressed to learn anything when you are first diagnosed or when problems arise. You might need to depend on relatives and friends to obtain medical knowledge and advocate for you until you are well enough to take over.

I can understand how some patients resist learning about the medical aspects of their illness. I remember how I felt when my microwave oven broke. My family uses our microwave all the time—for making popcorn, heating and reheating soups and meals, and warming my bed buddy, a rice-filled sock that can be used as a heating pad. One day, the touch pad went on the blink. Suddenly, and without apparent cause, the panel started flashing 88:88, and then the microwave went dead. This wasn't the first time it had gone on the fritz, but previously the unit restarted if I gave it a jiggle or waited a few minutes. So I jostled the microwave, touched every key on the control pad more times than I'd like to admit, unplugged it, and then plugged it back in. The blackened control panel and dead silence were infuriating. Aargh! I hadn't done anything wrong, as far as I could tell. Yet I couldn't heat up my lasagna for dinner. To make matters worse, I didn't know much about microwaves *and I didn't want to*. Like a toddler throwing a tantrum, my initial reaction was useless: "No fair! I want my microwave back, now!"

I could have chosen not to learn about the power supply of microwaves. This choice would have forced me to go through the hassle and expense of getting the oven repaired or replaced, or going without a microwave. Begrudgingly, I chose to obtain knowledge. I talked to a gentleman at an appliance repair shop who suggested a few likely possibilities to explain the problem and a few maneuvers to try. Armed with his instructions and a Phillips head screwdriver, I opened the box that housed the ground plug. The culprit was obvious: The plug's plastic casing had cracked, causing a short circuit. I then took the box, broken plug, and cord to the hardware store where a salesman showed me how to replace the ground plug and splice the old wires to the new one. After listening to his hints and warnings, I went home and tried it. It was easy. With my children cheering me on, I plugged in my microwave and, lo and behold, it worked! My bill? Three dollars and twenty-four cents. Reheated lasagna never tasted so good.

Obviously, there are important differences between dealing with illness and a broken microwave. I could have chosen not to learn anything about my microwave problem, a choice that would have had its downside but still would have been a reasonable option. Such an option isn't wise when talking about your health. Sure, you can put yourself in the hands of top doctors and nurses and trust them to take care of everything for you. But even the world's best physicians depend on information from you to do their job. Who can tell them what's happening in your body—your pain, numbness, fatigue, and weakness—better than you? Who, better than you, can help them make the best treatment decisions for you when there is no clear "right" answer? And who, better than you, can keep tabs on how you're doing between doctor visits? Your choice is this: What kind of control do you want

> Learn enough basic medical knowledge to help yourself and to help other people help you.

to have over your health? Over your life? You need to learn enough basic medical knowledge to help yourself and to help other people help you.

How much medical knowledge is enough? To start, ask your doctors and nurses what you need to know today: details about your specific medical condition, your treatments, and the warning signs and symptoms of problems. Over time, you'll fill in the gaps. You don't need to become a de-facto doctor who learns everything possible about your medical situation, and you don't need to learn everything at once. How much is enough depends upon your medical condition, your personal need for information, and your relationships with your physicians. At the very least, you need to be able to:

- understand what your doctors and nurses are saying to you,
- recognize any problems you are experiencing, and
- talk with your health-care team about your problems.

Obtaining medical knowledge is essential because *you* are the first line of defense against potential medical problems, unless you are in the intensive-care unit where you are hooked up to monitors and have nurses watching over you twenty-four hours a day. If something is happening in your body, you are the first one to experience it and be in a position to call for attention from people who can help. Knowledge helps you recognize a medical problem and respond in healthy ways.

How well do you understand your current medical situation?
How well can you care for your own medical needs? How active
a player do you want to be in making medical decisions about
your care and monitoring your progress between office visits?

Using Medical Terms

Medical knowledge begins with words. Even the simplest words can be troublesome in the setting of serious illness. Some patients go to great lengths to avoid saying the name of their disease. Using medical words can be your first step toward Healthy Survivorship because the act of saying a phrase changes how you feel about these words and what they mean. I remember how I got a charge out of referring to Ted as "my husband" in the weeks following our wedding. Using this new label for my sweetheart felt awkward in an exciting way and helped our recent marriage feel more real. Now, twenty-three years later, saying the words *my husband* is about as thrilling as mentioning the Cheerios I ate for breakfast, even though I'm still madly in love with him.

Whereas the romance and excitement of a new title are pleasurable, the emotional charge of medical terms can be terribly unsettling when adjusting to a new illness or injury. I'll never forget the staggering sadness I felt the first time I mentioned in conversation that I had an appointment with an oncologist. Now it doesn't bother me in the least. If anything, the term elicits positive feelings of respect and gratitude. And although undergoing a bone-marrow transplant would be an emotionally trying experience, I now can talk about the possibility of needing one in the future as if I were discussing an upcoming hair appointment. Using medical words helps me talk about emotional topics unemotionally when I need to. If something is so awful that you can't even say its name aloud, it has great power over you. Calling your disease and its treatment by their proper names gives you back some of that power. Listen to yourself when you talk with others. What words do you use to describe your condition? For example, do you say the medical name or do you say my "illness" or "little problem" or "situation"? By paying attention to your emotions when you use or hear medical words you gain insight into how you are doing.

Suppose you find it hard to use medical terms. What should you do? Children sometimes show us the simplest solutions to adult problems. I heard a story of a young girl who stood on her tiptoes in her bedroom and stared at her reflection in the mirror above her dresser, repeating, "Leukemia, leukemia, leukemia, leukemia . . ." Her father heard her voice, cracked open her bedroom door to peek, and asked in a puzzled voice, "What are you doing?" His daughter explained matter-of-factly, "I'm saying the name of your sickness until it doesn't scare me so much."

By talking about your "multiple sclerosis," "prosthesis," or "physical therapy," these words become part of your everyday vocabulary and don't trigger the same emotional response as they did the first few times you heard or used them in reference to yourself. Saying the words often diminishes their ability to trigger the unpleasant or disabling emotions of fear, shame, embarrassment, or sadness. Giving a humorous spin to emotionally charged medical terms may help you use certain words when, otherwise, you couldn't. A patient with colon cancer first talked about her illness by joking, "My cancer surgery helped me improve my punctuation. Now I use a semicolon!"

More than helping you adjust to the name of your illness, using medical terms gives you confidence and helps you adjust to the accompanying changes and challenges. I suspect that this phenomenon explains my husband's odd behavior when he was forty-nine years old. Most people over thirty tend to underestimate their age. Yet, during the months following his forty-ninth birthday, Ted answered "fifty" whenever people asked him his age. It was as if he were preparing for the notorious milestone by trying the age on for size and seeing how it felt before it really counted. His use of language helped make the transition comfortable. What's especially interesting about this story is that Ted was unaware that he was doing it until a student remarked, "Professor Harpham, why are you saying you're fifty? You're only forty-nine."

Words help you adjust to the reality of your illness because you know things in different ways. I knew my cancer diagnosis, rationally, before I really believed it was true. My sense of unreality was helpful during the initial crisis because it protected me from being overwhelmed by all the unexpected changes. But shock is a place to visit and not a good place to stay. In the long run, it is only when I am no longer dazed that I can act most effectively, make my life easier, and enjoy a sense of living most fully. Using emotionally charged medical terms in conversation, letters, or journal entries helped the different parts of me—my rational self and my emotions—get in step with each other. I remember the day after my diagnosis when I was being wheeled to radiology for a scan and a colleague came over and asked, "Wendy, what's going on?" Instead of sharing what I knew by saying something like "I have lymphoma" or "My doctors found (or the biopsy showed) lymphoma," I answered, "*They say*

I have lymphoma." I knew the lymphoma diagnosis but wasn't yet ready emotionally to say it was certain. Within days, as I began to know in my heart what I knew in my head, I made the transition to saying, "I have cancer," and in doing so began to accept on an emotional level the reality of my illness. How I talked about my cancer not only reflected my increasing readiness to accept it; my choice of words also helped me adjust at a pace that worked for me. Using medical terms and talking about your illness are ways you can help yourself adjust to a new normal.

The problem of language is bigger than the names of your illness and treatments. The whole world of medical terms can be a problem, making you feel alienated from those around you. A friend of mine who doesn't speak Spanish told me how scary it was to develop appendicitis while traveling in a remote region of Spain. Imitating the Spanish paramedics, she emphasized how the seeming frenetic pace of their language just heightened her anxiety and fed her imagination. I can imagine what it must be like for you if you don't have a medical background because I've had the experience of learning another language. I remember how my French teacher's speech sounded impossibly fast the first day of class. After I learned only a few words and phrases, however, her speech seemed slower and clearer even though it was exactly the same. I was amazed: A little familiarity with the foreign tongue made me hear it differently.

Your doctors and nurses use medical terminology to communicate to one another and to the allied health professionals with whom they work, such as physical therapists, dietitians, radiation therapists, social workers, and counselors. When you are familiar with the language of your illness, even if you don't yet know or understand much, you may feel less frightened by your situation or estranged from the people who can help you.

Is using these words helpful or harmful to you right now? In general, medical terms are beneficial if using them makes you feel brave, safe, empowered, confident, or more whole. These feelings may occur almost simultaneously with your first utterance of medical terms, or the positive feelings may wash over you only after a delay or after repeated use. Wait an hour or two, or even a couple of days, before you judge the full effect that your use of language is having on you. Using emotionally charged words in conversation empowers you if, and only if, you are ready to use them. If saying certain words or talking about a specific topic causes you great anxiety that lingers, you may not be ready yet.

Be forewarned that you may be ready to use medical terms and talk about certain topics before your friends and family members are. Judgment and trial and error will help you figure out when your use of medical language encourages others to adjust, or makes it harder for them to relate to you. Their comfort level with using or hearing medical terminology probably will change over time. Sometimes, bluntly telling loved ones that it helps you to talk about your illness will help them listen to you in a caring way. At the very least, it is better than having them unsure how to respond. Using medical terms is good when it helps things seem more real, connects you in healthy ways to the people around you who are important, and makes you feel better in some way.

How comfortable are you using medical terminology? The name of your disease? The names of your treatments? Right now, is it helpful or harmful for you to use medical words? When is using medical terminology helping you adjust?

The Power of Understanding Medical Terminology

The real power behind learning a new language comes not from making the words familiar to your ear but from understanding their meaning. Here's a story that illustrates the danger you face if you don't learn basic medical terms that apply to your illness. Picture a man who moves to a foreign country. Out of laziness or stubbornness, he refuses to learn anything about the local language or culture. Not surprisingly, he has a hard time making his needs known and tending to them. Warnings or advice expressed in the native tongue are useless. Whenever he develops a problem, his inability to communicate effectively leaves him vulnerable. Suppose this fellow is hungry one day. He sees a native pluck a berry and pop it in her mouth, gesturing for the stranger to try one. The man wonders if the berries are poisonous, tentatively sliding a berry in his mouth and biting down. When his teeth rupture the berry's firm skin, a sharp burst of acid on his tongue fuels his fear. He spits it out. The native is puzzled, and tries to explain, "Gooseberries—tart but nutritious. We eat them all the time." The foreigner doesn't trust the native, so he remains hungry and afraid; the native is unable to help him.

Just because you depend on the expertise of others to help diagnose and treat your medical problems doesn't mean you have to be a stranger in a foreign land. By learning a few technical terms and the basics about your medical condition, you'll make it easier for your doctors and nurses to explain to you what they are doing and why. And, since you'll be better able to discuss your concerns and needs with your health-care team, they'll be able to take better care of you.

Remember that different people learn languages at different speeds. My husband had a terrible time in his high-school French classes. The language remained unintelligible for a long time, and he struggled to get through the three years of required foreign language. Thirty years later, he still wakes up in a cold sweat every once in a while because he's having a nightmare about flunking his French final exam! Despite his difficulties in high school, he actually did learn enough to pass all his French exams. Don't be embarrassed or discouraged if it takes a lot of time and effort to learn a little medicine. It will come.

Who is helping you learn the medical terms used to discuss your illness? How are you going about learning them?

Medical Knowledge Minimizes Miscommunication

Miscommunications and misunderstandings cause trouble, especially when dealing with health issues. Miscommunications are minimized when you understand the lingo. Imagine a curious patient (this happens all the time, by the way) who can't resist peeking at her X-ray report while carrying it from the radiology department to her doctor's office for her routine checkup. She almost faints, assuming she has cancer when she sees the top line that reads, "R/O cancer." Actually, the patient may be perfectly healthy and her X ray perfectly normal. "R/O cancer" is short-hand for "Rule out cancer," a heading for an X-ray request and subsequent report that is used in certain cases even when the doctor's suspicion that the patient has cancer is extremely low, but the possibility of cancer has to be ruled out because of a particular symptom. As another example, when one of my friends was diagnosed with leukemia, she asked her physician to send her a copy of the letter that he had sent to the insurance company. She became panic-stricken when it arrived and she read, "The patient's brother is a one-antigen mismatch." The test result indicated good compatibility for all but one marker, more than enough for the transplant. Concluding erroneously that his marrow was not usable, she despaired of getting the bone-marrow transplant she needed to save her life.

This sort of eavesdropping on information not intended for you is an invitation to miscommunication. Similar problems occur when you overhear your physicians talking on the telephone or to their colleagues outside your exam room. I suggest you not read or listen to information not intended for you. When you do—by accident or on purpose—discuss with your physicians what you've learned. Misunderstandings occur in direct conversations, too, as illustrated by the joke about the patient who complains of ear pain. His doctor diagnoses an ear infection and writes out a prescription, complete with instructions. The patient returns to his doctor three days later, "My pain is worse, and now I'm deaf in that ear." The doctor whisks out an otoscope and looks in the patient's ear. "Oh, my! You have six pills stuffed in your ear canal." The patient answers, "But, Doc, I did everything you said to do," handing over the instruction sheet that says to take one pill twice a day for ear pain. It's not funny when such things happen in real life, and they do.

Even when no serious physical harm occurs, miscommunications can cause emotional distress. For instance, a nurse tells a hospitalized patient whose IV isn't working, "You've lost your access." The patient begins crying, thinking that she can't get any more treatments when, in fact, "lost your access" means that the intravenous line isn't working and she needs a new one, and not that she's lost her right or ability to be treated. Medicine is complex, and miscommunications will happen even under the best of circumstances. If you learn the language used to discuss your medical condition and treatments, you minimize miscommunications that can lead to bodily harm or emotional distress.

If you read or hear information that was not intended for you, do you check what you've learned with your doctor?

Medical Knowledge Offers Motivation

By helping you understand what is happening, medical knowledge may help you stay motivated. After the neck surgery that led to the diagnosis of my first recurrence, my physician ordered a specialized CT scan of my head. In order to obtain the best image, I was placed flat on my stomach with my head facing forward. At first, I giggled, feeling like the human cannonball in the circus. The humor of the situation faded quickly as the technician instructed me to hold still in this uncomfortable position forever (or was it just fifteen minutes?). My surgical site began throbbing and the back of my neck cramped up. The discomfort let loose my imagination about what pain might accompany my upcoming treatments. I'd always calmed myself during other uncomfortable procedures by talking to whoever was around or by doing the Lamaze breathing exercises that had enabled me to deliver all my babies naturally. (I don't want to brag, but you might better appreciate my pain tolerance if I mention that my son weighed over ten pounds!) Unfortunately, the radiology suite was not like any labor and delivery room. While I was lying in the scanner, my breathing was directed by the disembodied voice over the loudspeaker that commanded, "Take a deep breath. . . . Hold it. . . . Breathe. . . . Take a deep breath. . . . Hold it. . . ." Lamaze was out of the question.

Medical knowledge made the difference. I knew that high-quality X-ray pictures would help my doctors assess my current situation. I also knew that if I moved, the pictures wouldn't be as clear. We might lose useful information that would help us make wise treatment decisions, or I might have to go through the procedure again. More than I wanted to be out of that machine, I wanted my doctors to have the information they needed to help me. Knowing the benefits of high-quality scans helped me to change my perception of the discomforts and gave me the necessary stamina to endure them.

If you are having a difficult time dealing with the demands of being a patient, find out more about what's being done to you and why it is being done, or what is being expected of you and why. Your courage and strength may increase when you know what to expect and what you can do to make your experience more tolerable. Courage and calm arise from an appreciation of the value of these tests, procedures, and treatments. Most important of all, this knowledge can build your trust in the health-care team, an essential element of Healthy Survivorship.

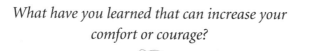

*What have you learned that can increase your
comfort or courage?*

Resolving Unfounded Fears

Obtaining knowledge also helps you by resolving fears based on myth or misinformation. This is true in any situation. Imagine two young brothers who are camping in their backyard and awaken to a scratchy noise outside their tent. The five-year-old boy freezes, imagining a purple three-headed monster poised to enter their tent and tear them to pieces. The eleven-year-old doesn't believe in imaginary monsters so doesn't share this fear. Yet he, too, is paralyzed by the sound as he pictures a hungry bear sniffing in search of something (or somebody!) to eat for a midnight snack. The two brothers huddle together, their imaginations spinning increasingly terrifying endings. Too afraid to peek outside, they never see the branch of a tree brushing up against their tent.

The boys are rescued when their dad comes to check on them. All three laugh about how the boys were scared of a twig. They readily admit that it wasn't funny at all before their dad "saved" them. This story demonstrates two important ideas: First, fear can keep you from information that will resolve your fear and, second, one piece of accurate information can tame a variety of fears.

Patients who don't learn about their condition or treatments unwittingly avoid learning about changes that are *not* problems and about problems that are *not* likely to occur. Medical knowledge eliminates (or, at least diminishes) the fear surrounding normal, expected, or healthy changes related to your illness. Healthy Survivors don't waste energy being afraid of big nothings. For example, Adriamycin is a chemotherapy drug that causes red urine. Not knowing this, the average cancer patient taking Adriamycin may fear something awful is happening when he sees red in the toilet bowl. Advance warning allows these people to feel a certain comfort because they now associate the crimson with their healing medicine. Simple medical knowledge transforms the reality of red urine from a source of fear to one of comfort.

Medical knowledge eliminates fears of events that are unlikely or impossible, too. When I developed sparkles and wavy lines in my visual field the night after receiving my first dose of chemotherapy, a host of diagnoses came to mind, the most frightening of which were lymphoma of the brain and impending stroke. I called my oncologist, who suspected an optic migraine related to the chemotherapy. While giving me instructions on what to do, he mentioned offhandedly, "By the way, your type of cancer rarely, if ever, spreads to the brain." With those few words, my level of anxiety dropped. The visual symptoms resolved soon thereafter and never recurred. Even if they had persisted, and even if I'd needed to undergo a full evaluation, my fear of brain metastases (lymphoma spread to my brain) would have been decreased, as well as any emotional discomfort related to that particular fear.

As you jump through diagnostic and treatment hoops, your body may respond in ways you've never experienced. You may have new aches and pains, weird skin changes, or who knows what. Without knowledge, your imagination is free to consider all sorts of wild possibilities. Obtaining sound knowledge will help resolve any fears that are based on myth or misinformation.

What fears about your condition have you kept secret and not shared with anyone? What myths have you been able to dispel with sound knowledge?

Resolving Minor Medical Problems

Basic medical knowledge can help tame your fear when minor problems develop, too. A middle-aged man from my cancer support group learned this the hard way. He told us how he'd developed a cough soon after completing successful radiation therapy for a localized lung cancer. Unaware of the variety of possible causes of the cough and understandably afraid that his cancer was back, he delayed medical evaluation. When he finally got tired of coughing (actually, I think his family's nagging wore him down), he saw his physician and was found to have a benign and treatable condition related to his recent treatments. Obtaining knowledge about the source of his cough ended his weeks of physical and emotional distress and led him to conclude, "I wish I'd bucked up and gone in earlier."

When dealing with illness, you can't expect your course to be perfectly smooth from diagnosis through recovery. Minor problems and setbacks occur even if, ultimately, you do fabulously well. Expecting minor problems, recognizing them, and knowing what to do when they occur will make your life much easier. Obtaining medical knowledge helps tame fears precipitated by new symptoms by giving you many possible explanations to think of, including hopeful ones. Discussing your symptoms with your health-care team gives you access to means of minimizing the pain, debility, and loss due to minor treatable medical problems.

*How often do you keep secret a new symptom because you are
afraid of what it might be?*

Learning about Signs and Symptoms

What about the signs and symptoms of medical problems you are not
having now? Do you need to learn about them? Wouldn't you be better off
sparing yourself the additional stress of worrying about potential disasters? As for those problems you are not likely to develop, why get yourself
in a tizzy, even if only for a moment? You need to know them for the same
reason you are instructed by an airline stewardess about the location of
the emergency exits before every takeoff. Statistically speaking, when you
fly you will never use an emergency exit. Yet airlines make the effort to
educate you because emergencies *are possible*, even if only remotely so,
and the information *is vital* in the event of an emergency landing.

You need to learn about signs and symptoms of potential problems
because these are your body's way of signaling you about your medical
condition. Sometimes, the sign or symptom is simply providing information. When an incision looks fine but becomes itchy, the itchiness is a signal that your wound is healing. Other times, the signal is a warning.
When an incision becomes inflamed, it indicates that your wound is
probably infected. Obtaining knowledge about the warning signs and
symptoms of medical problems—what they are and what you should
do—helps decrease your anxiety and confusion about your condition.

Medical knowledge helps you read your body's signs and signals and
respond appropriately. *Any* change is a signal, especially if unexpected. A
signal can be an ache or pain, rash, swelling, cough. It can also be a difference in your usual energy, skin color, memory or concentration, weight,
or sleep cycle. Knowledge helps you evaluate your symptoms more
calmly, know which ones are warning signs, and respond appropriately.
Just like the emergency-room triage nurse who can do a quick assessment
of each patient and decide if the patient's problem needs immediate

attention, medical knowledge gives you a sense of whether your symptom signals a problem that is minor, serious, or potentially life threatening. The biggest advantage of being knowledgeable about signs or symptoms is that early intervention in problems or complications often improves your outcome. Hence, medical knowledge helps you deal with the uncertainty by increasing your chance of a safe journey and bolstering your

> Remember: You can know something without thinking about it all the time.

confidence in one. Once you learn what you need to learn, put the information in the back of your mind, where it can stay forever (unless you develop worrisome signs or symptoms).

How familiar are you with your body's signs and symptoms? Which ones are signals of potential problems?

The Value of Recognizing and Responding to Warning Signs

Look at the virtue of recognizing and responding to warning signs. A professional pickpocket approaches his first target of the day—an elderly woman. The thief gracefully slips his hand into the woman's open purse and, without causing so much as a single vibration, plucks out her wallet. Long after he disappears from the scene, she discovers the theft. The pickpocket then finds another potential victim. This time, his wrist catches on the strap and gives the purse a tiny jerk. The owner of the purse is talking on her cell phone and ignores the tug. Again, the thief gets away with his loot. The pickpocket now approaches a third woman from behind. As his hand dips into her purse, the woman happens to shift her weight and feels a subtle tug on her shoulder strap. She turns quickly, sees the robber, and screams. He drops the wallet and runs.

Without warning signs from your body, you would be oblivious to impending danger. Like the tug on the woman's purse strap, your symptoms are an opportunity. It's up to you to pay attention. Ignore warning signs, and you risk trouble. Everyone is wired differently. A symptom that is slightly annoying to one person may immobilize another. Understand

New symptoms are your friends.

that the problem is *not* how much anxiety you feel, or whether the degree of your fear is justified. The problem is the temptation to downplay worrisome symptoms, ignore them, or explain them away without getting needed medical attention.

New symptoms are your friends, but they can help you only if you pay attention to them and respond appropriately. Ask your doctors and nurses to teach you how to recognize signs and symptoms and what to do when you detect something new. Pamphlets and books written by medical professionals may be helpful, too. If you read information conflicting with your own physicians' advice, discuss the discrepancy with them.

How do you respond to new symptoms?

Symptoms That Persist or Come Back

When your symptom has been evaluated and treated, yet doesn't improve or improves and then returns, you might be reluctant to go back to your physician. Giving up is a mistake. If a leaky faucet continues to drip after your plumber said he fixed it, you'd get the plumber back or get a new plumber. Your persistent symptom merits reevaluation and retreatment, as if it were a new problem. The medical evaluations and treatments should stop only after you and your physicians conclude that the diagnosis is as clear as possible, and that everything is being done to make things better. After treatment, a persistent or recurrent symptom can be a clue that your diagnosis was missed, your treatments aren't working well, or you've developed a new problem. Hang in there! However long it takes and no matter how many treatments are required to get you well, keep working with your doctors.

What if you suspect that your treatments are incorrect or your doctor is incompetent? You might be right! Or, you might be wrong and simply have a problem that is not responding to the treatments that usually work well. The most efficient way to put your concern to rest is to get a second opinion from another physician, preferably one not affiliated with the first. You have a right to good care, and second opinions are a routine part of good medical care, especially when things are not going smoothly. A second opinion will either reassure you (and your doctor) that your current treatments are on target, or you will learn of a better treatment approach. Either way, second opinions help you and your doctors work together toward a common goal: getting you better.

Are you keeping your physicians informed of persistent or new symptoms or concerns?

Learning about Aftereffects

Aftereffects are changes and problems that occur after completion of treatment. Based on true stories, let me tell you about two women who underwent removal of their axillary (armpit) lymph nodes as part of their evaluations for breast cancer. After completing their cancer treatments, Sally chose to read her pamphlet about the possible aftereffect of lymphedema, a swelling of the arm that can lead to cosmetic deformity, pain and disability, and life-threatening infection. Meredith filed away her information sheet on lymphedema, wanting to avoid dealing with any issues and emotions that she felt she didn't have to. One night, they each noticed pink puffiness around their index fingernails where the cuticle was torn slightly. Sally recognized the redness as a sign of possible early infection, called her doctor, and was started on antibiotics within an hour. A few days later, her finger was back to normal. Meredith went to bed, unaware of the significance of the redness. She awakened in the early morning with fever and chills, and her arm was swollen with painful red streaks. A course of intravenous antibiotics cured the skin infection but not before the lymphatic vessels in her arm were permanently damaged, leaving her with a chronically swollen arm.

Obtaining knowledge about aftereffects allows you to take steps to prevent or minimize them, recognize problems early (when they are usually most treatable), and work as a partner with your doctors and nurses to intervene when possible. Learning about her risk enabled Sally to make timely decisions about her health. As Meredith learned the hard way, ignorance is *not* bliss when it means closing the window of opportunity to improve your health during and after recovery.

How well-informed are you about aftereffects?

Screening Tests

The bad news is that you are not immune to other medical problems during and after treatment. The good news is that in many cases screening studies done at routine checkups can alert you and your physicians to silent conditions that require medical attention. If you feel fine and a screening test tips your doctors off to a problem, you've caught it as early as possible. Don't panic if a screening test shows a worrisome change because all it means is that you *might* have a problem. Further testing may show the screening test result was a false positive, and you are fine.

Make sure you don't ignore symptoms that develop weeks or months after a normal screening test. It is a mistake to assume your symptoms are insignificant since your recent test results were normal. For one thing, medical tests only provide information about your condition on the day the tests were done. You may have developed detectable changes after the test. For another, even if your screening test was done this morning, the screening test may have been a "false negative," missing your problem. It is the *combination* of (1) screening tests and (2) your knowledgeable attention to signs and symptoms that comprises a powerful two-prong warning system that provides you with opportunities to respond in positive ways.

How do you respond to symptoms that persist or develop after
a normal screening test?

Risk Factors

*Risk factors: circumstances, conditions, or behaviors
that increase your chances of developing a certain
medical problem.*

As with any nonmedical risk, what actually happens in your life is affected by both your risk due to factors beyond your control and your response to your risk factors that are within your control. If you live in a high-crime neighborhood, you can take steps to decrease your *overall risk* of being robbed such as locking your doors and windows, leaving on a few lights when you leave your house, and installing an alarm system linked to your police department.

Let's suppose that, despite your efforts, your home is burglarized. You and others may be tempted to conclude, "Why bother taking precautions if I can be robbed anyway?" Although you can't guarantee safekeeping, you bother because your efforts *can* make the difference between having and not having your valuables. The locked doors and bright lights will deter many criminals. Any thieves who manage to break into your home will set off the alarm and, probably, get caught or run away before they can do much damage. In a similar way, learning about your medical risks and what you can do to minimize them can mean the difference between being a victim and a Healthy Survivor.

Link your knowledge of risk with positive action. Some of the medications in my chemo cocktail, as well as the chemo-induced menopause, put me at increased risk of osteoporosis, a thinning of the

Bad news becomes good news when it empowers you.

bones. In light of these and other risk factors, my physicians prescribed calcium supplements. When screening tests a few years later showed osteoporosis, my physicians prescribed additional prescription medication. Today, my bone scans are much improved, my risk of bone fracture is much lower, and I have a lot less reason to worry. Knowledge combined with action transforms distress to challenge, and panic to energy toward healing. When talking about medical information, bad news becomes good news when it empowers you.

What are your risk factors? What can you do to decrease your overall risk?

Celebrating False Alarms

When you are knowledgeable about the medical aspects of your illness—signs, symptoms, aftereffects, and risk factors—you may end up having more false alarms. After all, you will notice changes that you otherwise might have missed or thought were insignificant. You may end up going to your doctor for lumps or skin changes that turn out to be nothing important. It is this possibility of false alarms that leads many people to conclude that "ignorance is bliss."

As with any warning system, you need to take alarms seriously. Think about false medical alarms the way you think about fire drills. You may be inconvenienced by a fire alarm that turns out to be just a routine test of the system. But, if the alarm signals a real fire, you'll be glad you took it seriously and followed the directions for escape. In terms of medical false alarms, unless you have some magical guarantee that a sign or symptom is due to something that doesn't need medical attention, a false alarm is a small price to pay for the possibility of protecting your health or saving your life.

I can understand why you might not be thrilled after responding to a false alarm. One of my patients called my office, panicked about seeing blood in her stool. She came in, and I did an examination. Her stool was red, but it wasn't blood. When I questioned her about her food intake the previous evening, she suddenly remembered that she'd eaten a big bowl of cherry Jell-O. She burst out crying. "I'm so embarrassed. I'd feel better if you'd found a tumor rather than my dessert." But I was relieved, telling her how happy and proud I was that she had shown the good sense to come in, and thanking her for what was ultimately a humorous story for us both.

You can't live retrospectively. You can only live in the present, choosing your responses to today's signs and symptoms without knowing the outcome of your evaluation until you've been through it and received the results. False alarms are the price of not missing a real warning. Pursuing a false alarm can be expensive, uncomfortable, inconvenient, even risky. Sometimes the results are embarrassing or funny. Until medicine is perfect (and that won't happen any time soon), if you try to avoid false alarms, you'll be taking the risk of missing opportunities to prevent problems or fix them easily.

Focus on the many good sides of false alarms. First of all, you got good news. Celebrate! A false alarm is an emotional reminder of how well you are doing. And, false alarms can reinforce the idea that things can turn out fine even if some signs and symptoms are worrisome. See your good news as your reward for doing the right thing and responding appropriately to the warning sign. When I've had false alarms, I've tried to focus on how fortunate I am to be relieved of another medical problem with all its associated stress, expense, and uncertainty. "If that biopsy had shown cancer again, I'd be trying to make a treatment decision now instead of going off to the movies." False alarms can be a good part of Healthy Survivorship.

In the process of responding to warning signs or undergoing screening tests, you might find out about terrible medical problems that are looming on the horizon and are unstoppable even with the best of today's science and technology. Hard as you try, you may find it impossible to see any redeeming value to knowing about them. Certainly in these situations, ignorance is bliss, isn't it? Not for me. Ignorance is not bliss if it means taking the risk of sacrificing useful information. Sometimes bad news that seems totally unhelpful now turns out to be useful later. Although the news may be upsetting at first, and although I may not like my choices for responding to the news, I will always have choices. In chapter 7, I'll talk about using

> Ignorance is not bliss when it means closing windows of opportunity to improve your situation.

unpleasant emotions in ways that help you deal with whatever crisis or challenge you are facing, and letting go of emotions that only hurt you.

How seriously do you take alarms? How do you feel when you find out a warning signal was a false alarm? How do you celebrate false alarms?

Treatments

Obtaining sound and complete knowledge about your medical condition is one step toward becoming a Healthy Survivor. Once you know what your problems are, you are in a position to learn about possible solutions—treatments. A treatment is an intervention intended to help you. It can be a medicine, a procedure, or a method. It is anything you do or that you have done to your body to help you get better or feel better in some way. If you are going to help your physicians know which treatment matches your needs and goals the best, you have to know what each treatment is, and what it isn't. Even if you don't want to participate in any of the treatment decisions, learning about your treatments will help you deal with them. The rest of this chapter discusses how to judge information about medical treatments so that you weigh your choices wisely.

Choosing a course of treatment is hard when your physicians present various options. The decision can be even harder when your nurses, family members, and friends, as well as books and Internet Web sites offer a variety of solutions for all your ills. You may find yourself inundated with answers every which way you turn. What do you do with all this information, much of which is contradictory? How do you decide what risks to take, which people to trust, and what sacrifices to make in hopes of getting better? The answer begins with knowing how to compare the information you have about each of your treatment options.

Since all medical knowledge is not the same, you need a method of categorizing the facts and advice, especially information about treatments. You need something like a coin separator, one of those boxes that sort your pocket change. In the bottom of the box is a series of vertical tubes arranged snugly one against the other to catch coins. A slim tube for dimes abuts a slightly larger tube for pennies, and so on for the nickels and quarters. If you close your eyes and drop your coin into a slit at the top of the box, your coin will roll down and drop into the proper tube according to size. In essence, the box will determine for you the value of the coin. Just as a coin separator helps you know the value of each coin, an understanding of the differences between the various types of information helps you know whether a tidbit of information or piece of advice is worth a little or a lot. You will know how much confidence you should place in the various recommendations from your health-care team, other medical resources, and nonmedical sources such as the mass media, family, friends, and even strangers.

How do you decide how much weight to give a piece of information?

Sources of Information

What do I mean when I say that not all knowledge is the same? What are these different types of knowledge? Think about the following two scenarios: Imagine you receive a telephone call with a prerecorded message from a large real estate company saying "Congratulations! You are a winner!" Would you jump up and down with glee? Then again, imagine you hear the exact same message from the office of your dentist, a fun-loving guy who holds contests, such as awarding a gift certificate to the patient who best predicts the weight of his receptionist's new baby? I suspect you would have a different response to the same announcement. As a more relevant example, consider an article that announces a novel treatment for your disease. Would it make any difference if you saw this breaking news alongside a story documenting sightings of Martian invaders in a tabloid? What if the article was in a recent issue of the well-respected *New England Journal of Medicine*? Healthy Survivors know which sources provide reliable medical information.

For each of your treatment choices, what or who is the source of your information?

Reliable Science-Based Sources

Your physicians and nurses are your primary source of medical information. Not only do they provide facts and offer advice; they also can help you evaluate information you've obtained elsewhere. Articles, books, pamphlets, and Web sites discuss your illness with respect to the average patient, not you. Only a physician who has reviewed your particular situation can discuss if and how information pertains to you.

Nurses and allied health professionals such as nutritionists, radiation therapists, and physical therapists may have much to offer in their areas of expertise. But when it comes to choosing a course of treatment, keep in mind that they do not have the same medical background or perspective as your specialist. When you are weighing options, what nurses and allied health professionals *can* offer is helpful insight into other patients' experiences with the various treatments. Once you make a treatment decision, these professionals can offer practical advice about preparing for and getting through treatment. Be sure you share with your physicians what you've learned from your discussions with other health-care professionals.

Books and articles can be helpful or harmful. First, check the date of publication. Outdated material can make your situation appear bleak when in fact you have good treatment options and reason to be hopeful. Updated information about older options and novel treatments can shift the equation for you when deciding on a treatment course. Try to use materials that have been published within the last year or so, and always share what you've learned with your doctors.

Evaluating an author's ability to present accurate and up-to-date information isn't as straightforward as evaluating publication dates. University- or government-sponsored publications written by medical doctors tend to be less biased and provide high-quality science-based information about treatment. Some publications by pharmaceutical companies, nonprofit support organizations, and individual survivors are superb resources. Once again, your specialist can give you feedback on the usefulness of this information in your particular case. Web sites pose their own challenges; as with printed publications, those sponsored by universities and government agencies tend to be less biased and to provide high-quality information. However, some sites operated by physicians are misleading or dangerous, and some sites operated by nonmedical survivors are excellent. A few criteria will help you assess the quality of a site.

Tips for Evaluating Web Sites

- Origin: Is the site produced or sponsored by an academic center, government agency, pharmaceutical company, private-sector organization, physician, or nonphysician survivor or family member?
- Publication date: Is the site revised and updated regularly, and is outdated material removed from the site?
- Reputation: Does your oncologist feel this site is a reputable resource?
- History: How long has the site has been online? Has it stood the test of time?
- Awards: Has the site received awards for quality from independent reviewers or agencies?
- HON certification: Does the site claim to follow the codes of conduct of the "Health on the Net Foundation," a certification that suggests but does not guarantee quality?
- Conflicts of interest: Does the source of funding pose any potential biases for the material presented? If supported by a business organization or pharmaceutical company, it is better if funded by "Unrestricted Educational Grants."
- Contact information: Can you contact and communicate with the producers, editors, and contributing authors of the site? If not, this is a red flag.

Reputable science-based resources discuss treatments based on a long tradition of scrutiny and usage in conventional settings, or, more recently, evidence-based studies. If you read in a nonmedical magazine of a treatment that interests you, the next step is to see what the scientific literature has to say about this treatment. Medical librarians can help you do this. Or, you can ask your doctors, nurses, or someone with an interest in medical research to help you find out more. Whenever you come across material that is affecting how you are feeling about your care or what you are doing, run the information by your physicians. This gives them an opportunity to provide feedback on the information and helps them understand where you are coming from.

Anecdotal Information

In addition to knowing something about the source of information, it helps when you have an understanding of the difference between information obtained through anecdotes, observations, and science. Knowing the basis of each particular piece of information about your illness and treatment helps you weigh the strength of the conclusions and subsequent advice, and find your way to the best medical care possible.

Anecdotes come in different forms. Hearsay is an undocumented tale, a rumor, or an individual's version of what happened. Hearsay is one person saying "I heard that gobbledygook is good for your medical problem." The information may or may not be true, and may or may not be applicable to you. Another type of anecdote is someone's personal belief about a treatment. More than just sharing the news that the treatment is an option, he appears convinced that the treatment could fix your problem without presenting any evidence. The passion and confidence with which he presents his ideas may be compelling, and the treatment he is recommending may be appealing, too. But he is asking you to trust him without proof of any sort. The theory behind the effectiveness of the treatment may be true or false. The treatment may be helpful, harmless, or harmful to you. If you catch yourself seriously considering a treatment recommended by someone other than your physicians, ask yourself, "How does this person know it works? How do I know that this belief isn't misguided or mistaken?" Healthy Survivors recognize when they are tempted to try something just because it sounds good.

Still another type of anecdote is one that describes someone else's personal story. Think about how you feel when you hear or read about someone who is cured of the same illness you have. Let's say your long-time buddy from high school tells you that his Aunt Matilda was cured of the same disease by taking some particular treatment. Wanting the same outcome, you may feel connected to Aunt Matilda, but to base your medical decisions on such an anecdote is to throw away your opportunity to choose the best treatment for you. How do you know that she really had the same disease? How do you know she was really cured?

Even anecdotes that are impeccably accurate should not necessarily be the basis of a treatment decision. Let's say you read a well-documented account of a patient who had your exact medical condition, and who was cured after following a macrobiotic diet as her only treatment. The article may sound highly scientific, and the facts may be indisputably true. Understandably, you might consider following the same macrobiotic diet because you want the same end result. The report tells you only one thing: what happened to this one patient. It does not tell you how or why the patient got better. Even if the patient's cure *was* due to the macrobiotic diet, her individual success still doesn't tell you anything about how the diet worked, why it worked, or, most important of all, if it could work for you. If this patient had purchased a lottery ticket and won five million dollars, would you buy a lottery ticket, quit your job, and expect to become a multimillionaire, too?

Chances are high that the macrobiotic diet was not responsible for the patient's cure and that something else about her situation enabled the good outcome. Many similar patients follow a macrobiotic diet and die of their illnesses. You won't find their biographies in the bookstores. Patients and their loved ones want to read of rescue and triumph. Stories of failure, although important, don't sell. The next time you are in a bookstore or library, scan the titles in the self-help and health sections. You'll see dozens of success stories and few books (I suspect, no books) of someone's failed approach.

It's easy to understand the allure of personal success stories. They appeal to your emotions, putting names and faces to the notion that you can get well. But, *choosing* a treatment based totally on anecdote has no place in Healthy Survivorship. One particular problem with anecdotes is when faith healers ask you to put total trust in their powers and abandon any other forms of treatment. Faith healers appear invincible, and it's because they've got their bases covered. If you get well, they take the credit. If your illness progresses, they can blame *you* for the failure, saying "You must have had doubts. It would have worked if you had put complete faith in me."

Anecdotes not only can lure you toward unwise treatment choices; they can also lead you away from effective treatments. For example, if you know of someone who had a serious complication after undergoing the same test being recommended by your doctors, you may be reluctant to proceed even though the test is relatively safe and provides information that is vital to helping you get well. Don't judge what will happen to you by anecdotes of what happened to others.

Although anecdotes about other patients' recoveries can't help you *choose* treatment, they do serve useful roles. For one, success stories may stimulate scientists to look further into a treatment approach, especially if many patients report similar outcomes. For another, anecdotes about a particular treatment may prompt you to find out more about it and see if it might be a good option for you. Last, *after* you've chosen a course of treatment with your doctors, hearing or reading about success stories of similar patients who did well can bolster your hope.

Use anecdotes in healthy ways. Avoid people who demand that you abandon effective treatments offered by reputable physicians and who encourage you to pursue a treatment whose value is based solely on anecdote instead. Recognize the limits and dangers of anecdotes when choosing your course of treatment. And after you've made your decision, take advantage of the benefits of positive anecdotes.

How do success stories affect your feelings about a particular treatment choice? How do anecdotes with bad outcomes affect you?

Observational Evidence

Observation is a type of knowledge obtained through your senses. Many ancient remedies work fairly well because they are based on meticulous observation. For example, early civilizations had healers who, after generations of trial and error, knew which specific herbs and roots could bring down a patient's fever and which acupuncture sites could help relieve pain due to a broken bone. The forerunners to some of our most effective modern treatments came to scientists' attention through observation. For example, the role of vitamin C in the prevention and treatment of scurvy was determined through the observation that shipmates long at sea remained safe from this fatal disease if they ate limes. Today, observations like these are recorded and analyzed by the best scientific minds and analytical computers, prompting researchers to propose theories on ways to improve on current therapies.

Observation is important and useful, yet it has serious limits. This lesson hit home for me as a child when a popular joke circulated around my school playground: A young boy with a trained frog says, "Jump!" and the frog leaps. The boy then cuts off one of the frog's legs and says, "Jump!" The frog jumps. He cuts off a second leg, and then a third, and each time the boy says, "Jump!" the frog rocks and wobbles, then pushes forward. Then the boy cuts off the frog's last leg and says, "Jump!" The frog sits. The boy yells louder and louder, "Jump! Jump!" but the frog doesn't move at all. The boy concludes, "When you cut off all four of a frog's legs, the frog goes deaf." The most accurate observations can lead to wrong conclusions.

Observation is not relegated to scientists or healers. You are familiar with information obtained from your personal experiences. Let's say a physician prescribes an antibiotic, and you develop a strange blurring of your vision. Upon describing your symptom to the prescribing physician, you might be told, "That's not a reported side effect of that antibiotic, so it must be due to something else." Suppose that a few years later you take the same antibiotic for a different infection, and you develop the same blurry vision. Your doctor still thinks that your vision problem must be due to something other than the antibiotic. Since you've experienced the same exact problem only after taking this particular medication, you feel certain they are related. What are you supposed to believe—your own observations or your doctor's word? Balancing your personal observation with known scientific information is challenging.

Observation is a passive method of obtaining information; conclusions are based on what is seen or measured. This is not the best system available to help you with your medical problems. Even the most astute observer cannot be sure when two things that occur together represent cause and effect, i.e., one thing causes another, such as when two sticks rubbed together cause a spark. The two events could happen together without one causing the other, such as when your ice cream melts and you get sunburned under a blistering sun (neither of these events causes the other). Or two events could happen together by simple coincidence, such as when my husband, Ted, "helped" his beloved Philadelphia Phillies by taking a deep breath at home, miles away from Veteran's Stadium where a batter was swinging his bat for a grand slam.

Observation cannot test or modify a hypothesis, or draw conclusions about cause and effect. For every observation that leads to successful treatments, hundreds or thousands of similarly engaging observations lead to failure when subjected to rigorous study. This is because observation alone cannot tell you how or why something happened or if it will happen again, let alone provide insights that help scientists improve upon the process. Healthy Survivors appreciate the value and the limits of knowledge based solely on observation and use information based on science whenever possible.

How often do you draw conclusions based on your observation alone? How often do you draw conclusions based on someone else's observation?

Scientific Evidence

Science is defined as knowledge derived from observation *and experimentation*. A relatively new approach to studying the world, science has been around for a few hundred years but its use has intensified exponentially in recent history. The job of modern-day investigational science is to test theories based on anecdote, observation, induction, and intuition. Using stringent criteria for accuracy and reliability, science *proves* theories to be true or false.

Science is the most advanced method we have to determine which treatments are effective and which are not. Treatments derived from scientific inquiry are called evidence-based medicine and, in general, offer you the most reliable therapies available today. These treatments have been proven effective in people. Scientists may not yet have explained how or why every treatment does or doesn't work, but their well-done experiments can tell you *how well* each treatment works.

Any treatment that reliably and effectively helps a particular medical problem can be proven to work through scientific studies. Even when a treatment sounds kooky, if it really cures illness, it will stand up to scientific inquiry. For example, suppose you discover that ingesting a specific mushroom cures a syndrome characterized by fever, sore throat, and painful swallowing, and you propose that the mushroom promotes such healing by inducing a peaceful state of mind. Although you believe that a mushroom-induced calm cures sore throats, scientists would offer a different theory: The mushroom contains an antibiotic. Now suppose that, after rigorous scientific study, the mushroom treatment is proven effective. The issue here is not whether or not the mushroom induces a healing tranquillity. It is that *science can describe and validate the mushroom's healing power in scientific terms.* Scientific experiments would support the theory that the mushroom contains a penicillin-like substance that reproducibly cures infections due to certain bacteria, and is a good treatment. If scientific studies showed no benefit to eating the mushroom (i.e., if patients who ate the mushroom had the same outcome as those who didn't) science would have disproved the notion that this particular mushroom is a good treatment for this illness.

How does this idea of science help you deal with your illness today? From a utilitarian point of view, science is a powerful tool that helps you gauge the effectiveness of each of your treatment options and hedge your bets in your favor. Healthy Survivors take advantage of available conclusive information about treatment options.

Types of Information

- *Anecdote*: information obtained from a story. Anecdotal information includes hearsay, personal vignettes, individuals' beliefs, well-documented case histories, and superstitions. Anecdotes all share an inability to allow you to draw conclusions about the cause of events, or how these events relate to you.
- *Observation*: information obtained through the senses. Observation includes your personal experience, the personal experiences of others, and methodical observation and documentation by experts. All observations share an inability to explain how or why something happens, how two things are related, or how you can improve the situation.
- *Science*: information obtained through the senses and experimentation. Science is the modern-day tool for revealing the truth about what things are, how they work, how well they work, and how to improve on the results. Information based on science is reliable and reproducible.

The Truth

Science is a tool with one purpose: to uncover the truth about physical matters. For example, if you found a yellow ring, you might want to know "Is it gold?" You could try to figure it out by rubbing the metal between your fingers or by holding it in front of your eyes and examining it closely. You might even bite it the way people did years ago to test for purity. Such crude observations leave you vulnerable to harvesting fool's gold. You discover the truth about the purity of your ring only by using scientifically proven methods that determine the exact composition of the metal.

Science seeks a truth that is independent of the person claiming to possess the truth. As long as the test is done properly, a lump of gold will prove to be gold no matter which individual runs the scientific test, and whether you test it in Texas or on the moon. In contrast, a nonscientific approach might claim that the test works, but only if a person with supernatural powers runs the test in a mystery-shrouded chamber.

Proving the truth about the nature of your medical problems may be infinitely more complicated than proving the identity of a precious metal, but the concept is the same. If your leg hurts, a physician can use skilled observation and experience to propose a likely diagnosis such as "I suspect you have a pulled muscle" or "You might have a broken bone." Not until you undergo sophisticated blood, X-ray, or biopsy tests can the truth be determined. Scientific tests enable you to know the true cause of your pain.

In addition to helping you identify what things are, science uncovers the truth about how things do what they do. Science helps you know if and how you can change the natural course of events. A scientifically proven medical treatment works because it taps into a reliable and repro- ducible truth about the process of illness and healing. You can expect it to work to its proven degree, no matter what particular doctor administers it to you and no matter where in the world you get it, as long as it is the same treatment delivered in the same fashion. A drug treatment doesn't depend on some mystical powers outside of the drug. And although the special- ized skills held by a few surgeons may affect the success rate of sophisti- cated surgeries, this advantage is a matter of *training and skill*, not mystical powers. Scientific research is the modern-day tool for seeking the truth about disease and healing. Science-based medicine is the modern- day tool for seeking the truth about how best to help patients like you.

What if you don't connect with science? Maybe you're wondering, "Do I have to accept that the scientific method is a better manner of proof than a nonscientific one? Isn't it possible that another healing system such as one based on unorthodox methods or faith alone might offer me a better healing system? Science doesn't have all the answers about my illness. My doc- tors certainly don't have all the answers." When you were young, your teachers and parents didn't have all the answers either. You listened to their insights and advice because what they knew *was* helpful to you. A healthy perspective on science takes into account how you accept and use science in other aspects of your life. Every time you board a plane, flick a light switch, or pick

> Scientific research is the modern-day tool for seeking the truth about disease and healing. Science- based medicine is the modern-day tool for seeking the truth about how best to help patients like you.

up a telephone, you are using scientific knowledge. You expect the plane to take off no matter which particular pilot is at the controls. You expect the light to go on no matter who flips the switch. You expect to hear recognizable words when you pick up the phone.

Scientific explanations also help you by clarifying what you can't control. People in primitive cultures did rain dances or offered animal sacrifices, believing that the subsequent weather reflected the effectiveness of their appeals to their gods. Today, you may listen to the weather report and decide to take an umbrella with you, knowing that you can't control the weather but you can prepare for the likely precipitation. Use science to help you affect things under your influence and to prepare for and respond well to those things beyond your control.

Do any treatments you are using depend on some special mysterious power of the practitioner?

Faith Alone

When science doesn't have all the answers you want or need, you may become interested in healing systems based on faith alone. Faith is a powerful force, and believers don't feel the need for scientific proof. If anything, some people feel that a demand for proof may weaken the ability of faith to heal. Faith is beyond science. So, why couldn't faith be the best choice for you? This is an excruciatingly complex and charged topic. I won't attempt to solve this problem, but instead give you a perspective

Don't turn your back on science when it has something valuable to offer you.

that encourages you to *use science to your advantage* whenever you are dealing with medical problems, big or small. You don't have to choose between trusting your body to science and having faith. If you believe in a higher being, you can pray as you are wheeled into the operating room at a high-tech surgery center. If you want to, you can try to help your recovery by visualizing your wound healing properly while complying with your doctor-prescribed medications and physical therapy. One of the keys to being a Healthy Survivor is using science to your best advantage and not turning your back on science when it has something valuable to offer you.

At times, though, science will demand a rejection of other belief systems that keep you from the tangible benefits of modern medicine. As mentioned earlier, certain faith healers may insist that you refuse all conventional medical care in order to receive healing from their prayers. As a Healthy Survivor, in addition to recognizing the benefits of science and technology, you have to be willing to reject a mode of healing that demands you abandon science when science has something to offer you. If you feel unsure, remember that, for hundreds and thousands of years, people who nurtured deep spiritual faith died of strep throat, childbirth, and appendicitis. Cancer was a near-certain death sentence. Think about why so many people today survive once-fatal diseases: science.

Science and the Art of Medicine

The *science* of medicine is different from the *practice* of medicine. Science is a system of knowledge based on observation and experimentation. Medicine is an art based on science. The problem is that sometimes good scientists are bad artists. It is not healing to be kept for hours in a cold reception area, anxiously awaiting an upcoming test. Neither is it healing to come home to a message on your answering machine such as "This is Dr. Smith. Your HIV test came back positive. Please call my office after the weekend to schedule an appointment." It is terribly distressing when your specialist threatens to dismiss you because you've indicated an interest in pursuing complementary therapies such as acupuncture, or requested a second opinion, or simply brought in a list of questions. Healing is far more difficult when, after informing you that your illness is unlikely to respond to treatment, your physician extinguishes all hope, saying "Go home and get your affairs in order. You have six months." When upsetting things like this happen, you are unhappy with the *art* of medicine as it is being practiced, not the science behind the art. Don't reject science when you feel mistreated by a medical system that seems to strip you of power or take away hope. Instead, find competent physicians who relate to you in healing ways. As a Healthy Survivor, learn how to make the system work for you so that you can take advantage of what science has to offer.

When you distinguish the *science* itself from the *people and system* that use the science to administer its treatments, you can get the best out of both science and medicine. In order to squeeze the most out of a system that doesn't always work well, you may need to make changes in the way you do things and/or in your expectations, as was discussed in chapter 3. You may do best to seek assistance in dealing with a particular physician who is a good scientist and who can help you get better but who is not a particularly good caregiver. What matters most is that *you* get the *best* of what is available in today's world. I hope that as you undergo treatment and recovery, talking frankly with your health-care team about what helps you (and what harms you) will teach those who are caring for you some lessons in the art of medicine. By offering feedback in a respectful way, you are helping yourself and your physicians' other patients.

Moving On

Now that we've talked about obtaining medical information, it is time to use this knowledge for one of the most important decisions you make on the road to Healthy Survivorship: choosing a course of treatment. The next chapter will help you organize information about treatment so that you can make wise decisions that also reflect your personal needs, goals, and desires.

Choosing Your Best Treatment

*T*ed and I came home from our powwow with my oncologist. While Ted went to take care of the kids, I shut myself in our bedroom and called my best friend to fill her in. "Pam, I know all of my treatment options, but I don't like any of them!"

Once you know the extent of your illness, the key issue boils down to this: What are you going to do about it? That's where treatment comes in. Treatment is an intervention intended to help you. It can be a medicine, a procedure, or a method. It is anything you do or that you have done to your body to help you get better or feel better in some way. How do you decide if one treatment is better for you than another? You need to know what each treatment is, and what it isn't. You need to know the truth about how the treatments are alike and how they are different. Given your particular situation, you need to figure out what you want from your treatment, what you need from your treatment, what you can expect, and what you can hope for. This all boils down to having the facts you need to answer the essential question: What is the best treatment for you?

In becoming a Healthy Survivor, choosing a course of medical treatment is one of those occasions when getting the best care requires a dispassionate decision about something inherently emotional. This chapter provides a framework for classifying and understanding all the different types of treatments aimed at your physical healing. I will specify when I am referring to treatments used by cancer survivors because, in a few instances, treatment for cancer is different than treatment for other diseases.

This chapter is different from all the others and may be harder to read. I've included this material for those of you who want to be actively involved with your doctors in making treatment decisions as well as those of you who are interested in pursuing self-prescribed or alternative therapies for treating your illness. My primary purpose is to make clear the fundamental advantages that the class of conventional therapy offers over other classes of therapies. My goal is to help you make informed decisions and get the best care possible.

As you will see, in order to talk about your treatment options, you'll have to sort through a host of complicated technical terms. I realize that, despite my efforts to keep it as simple as possible, this chapter can become overwhelming. Take heart. Read whatever sections feel comfortable. You may need to skip most of this chapter for now and come back to it later, after you've had some time to adjust to your illness or even after you've started treatments. That's okay. The information can help you get through your treatments and deal with future decisions. For many of you, what will help you most is just looking at the tables—so you can review the basic differences between conventional, investigational, and alternative treatments—and then moving on to chapter 7.

> If deciding on a course of treatment feels extremely stressful, remember: Making a wise decision now will help decrease your stress for the rest of your life.

For those of you who want to learn more about your treatment options, this chapter will teach you how various treatments are the same, and how they are different. Only when you understand the risks and benefits of each of your options, and the limits of what is known about each option, can you compare apples against apples and know when you are comparing apples against oranges. This knowledge will help you choose the treatment path that feels right for you—

whatever path that may be—and enjoy the confidence, peacefulness, and hope that come with making an informed decision.

Your Choice

A distraught friend came to me with a list of her treatment options and asked, "Wendy, what's *my* best choice?" I couldn't determine her best choice of treatment any more than I could predict which of my home-cooked meals she would enjoy most. What I *could* do was teach her how to compare her options, with the expectation that so informed she would recognize the best choice for her. I could describe each of her treatment options just as I could describe all the ingredients and spices used in the preparation of each dinner entree. And I could help her learn the pros and cons of each choice. I could even make suggestions, but in the end, she would have to make the final decision and live with the consequences. Indeed, after a few weeks of research and discussion, she felt confident of her decision.

When a safe and reliably curative treatment is available for your medical problems, your choice may be easy: Go for the cure. Paradoxically, when dealing with an imminently life-threatening problem for which only one treatment offers *any* hope, your choice may be easy, too. It's when you have multiple treatment options and your illness is not imminently life threatening, or when you've exhausted all treatments known to be effective, that it becomes hard to decide what to do.

What treatment route you take is your choice. No matter how strongly your physician favors a certain approach, you are the one who makes the final decision. You are the one who decides between receiving conservative or aggressive treatments, and between using conventional therapies or trying an investigational therapy. As long as you are conscious, you are the one who decides when it is time to let nature take its course. You are the one who has to deal with friends and family members who are suggesting you try alternative therapies. And, you are the one who lives with the consequences of your choices.

How do you go about making this momentous decision? The knowledge-hope-action approach to Healthy Survivorship guides you to learn enough about your treatment options to work with your physicians in determining the best treatment approach for you. You don't have to become a medical expert about treatments any more than you'd need to become a gourmet cook to make a wise choice when presented with an array of exotic entrees. In most cases, Healthy Survivors base their treatment decisions on the advice of either their longtime trusted physician or, after spending time and energy consulting with various specialists, they follow the expert recommendation of one or more of them. On occasion, patients need (or prefer) to steer the course of their treatments. In most cases, your involvement falls somewhere in between, with you and your physicians having a dialogue, working together to chart a course for you. No matter what the case, it helps you if you have some understanding of the different types of treatment options and how to choose from among them. You are helping your health-care team take care of you, too, when you are knowledgeable about your treatments.

Over and over I hear stories of intelligent, well-motivated people who make terrible treatment decisions. While suffering the consequences, they say, "If only I'd known *then* what I know *now* about my treatments." It's sad. Unlike these people, you can make informed decisions about your treatment at every phase of illness and recovery. You can enjoy the confidence that comes with knowing you are doing the best you can, so you don't ever have regrets, no matter what happens.

Who can help you learn about your treatment options?
Who can help you compare your options?

Treatment Options

What becomes painfully obvious as you try to compare medical treatments is that they are a hodgepodge of choices with overlapping definitions, varying levels of proven validity, and ever-present uncertainty. In addition, how specific information is presented to you can affect how you interpret the facts. For example, you'd probably feel different depending on if your doctor said "This treatment is highly toxic and may not work" or "This treatment is aggressive and offers you the best chance of getting better." Both descriptions of the particular medical treatment may be equally accurate, yet might lead you to different decisions.

On top of everything, dry facts and statistics about treatments are superimposed on the mysteries of illness and healing. When the outlook appears certain, the unexpected still can happen, for better or for worse. Occasionally patients with "incurable" diseases or horrible medical complications surprise everyone and do well; and occasionally patients with highly curable diseases die even when everyone does everything right. The stress is enormous when you have complex or tough-to-treat medical problems. Given the ever-present risks and uncertainty, especially if your illness is life-threatening, any discussion of treatment options goes beyond rational thinking and taps into your belief system about healing, your emotional need for comfort and hope, and your spiritual faith.

With medical treatments being a confusing medley of options laced with uncertainty, how can you possibly make wise decisions? In today's complex and imperfect medical system, is it even possible? The answer is "Yes!" You can make wise decisions based on a sound framework for understanding and comparing all your treatment options, each one set against the others. Since you are unique, obtaining sound knowledge about treatment allows you to work with your physicians to find the best path *for you*.

The Red Flag of Multiple Explanations

When discussing a problem, the persistence of conflicting explanations and solutions is a red flag: The absolute truth is not known or a universally reliable solution has not yet been found. Wherever mystery persists, multiple explanations flourish. Imagine a family heirloom is missing—a gold watch, for instance. The members of your family may come up with a variety of theories of what happened to it. Each explanation may engage you to one degree or another and prompt certain actions such as searching under the car seats or in the laundry room. As long as the fate of the timepiece remains a mystery, a variety of both reasonable and far-fetched explanations can be entertained. Once you find the watch, the equation changes: All explanations other than the truth are meaningless. If the watch is found in the bottom of a dresser drawer, for instance, everyone would abandon the theory that it was buried with Aunt Susie. This notion is the basis of the riddle "Why do you always find what you're looking for in the last place you look?"

In any situation where you have a reliable solution or you know the truth, you are not tempted by a variety of conflicting explanations or answers. How does this idea relate to your health? Patients and their healers have long wanted to uncover the truth about safe and reliable ways to relieve physical suffering. For most of today's curable ills, after science developed reliable methods of diagnosis and treatment, the panoply of alternative therapies for these conditions fell into disuse. Few people today would turn to alternative methods of healing for a broken arm, appendicitis, bleeding ulcer, or cleft lip. Modern medicine offers safe and reliable solutions for these problems. It wouldn't make sense to look elsewhere. On the other hand, many patients today are turning to alternative methods of curing osteoarthritis, multiple sclerosis, Parkinson's Disease, allergies, and even the common cold because, despite advances in medicine, these problems still are hard to cure. Until science provides reliable answers for particular problems, healers and patients dealing with these problems will continue to engage in all sorts of explanations and treatments.

Pay attention to what science *does* know about your illness.

Regarding medical treatment for your particular condition, when conventional scientists don't all agree on treatment approaches you can assume that better answers are waiting to be found. Until that time, alternative treatments for your condition will abound. Your job is to get the best treatment you can. Science has better answers for some medical ills than others. Unfortunately, science may not have good answers for all your medical problems. In order for you to get the best care, pay attention to what science *does* know about your illness even if science hasn't explained or found treatments to cure you easily, if at all.

Unique Healing

You can enjoy the benefits of modern-day medicine as part of your personal healing program. As discussed in chapter 2, your healing is a complex process that depends on more than just receiving the medical treatment having the best statistical record of cure. Elusive elements such as your individuality, spirituality, relationships with your health-care team and caregivers, faith, and your will to live all play roles, too, not only in your quality of life but also, I believe, in your response to treatment and your length of life. Thankfully, researchers are starting to make efforts to look at these issues in scientific ways. Admittedly, science is only scratching the surface of the many mysteries surrounding *your* unique experience of illness and healing, but researchers are pushing to devise tailored cures for each patient.

The problem for you is that you need answers today. When you have cancer or another serious illness, you don't have the luxury of waiting for science to find better answers before you decide what to do. As a Healthy Survivor, take the best available scientific information based on populations of other patients, and, with your physicians, figure out what might work best for you today.

Comparing Apples Against Oranges

Ideally, when considering your treatment options, you compare apples against apples by comparing one well-studied treatment against another. This can be difficult, if not impossible, because treatments, even the various conventional treatments, have been studied scientifically to different degrees. While some of your options have been well investigated and proven effective for patients like you, others have little or no scientific data available for review. To complicate matters, newer treatments may offer unique benefits but have short track records because they are so new. What all this means is that, unfortunately, you may be forced to compare apples against oranges when choosing treatments for your disease.

> Compare apples against apples when choosing.
> Know when you are comparing apples against oranges.

Knowing that you are doing so will help you. As a general rule, give priority to treatments that have been proven effective or are based on sound science unless there are compelling reasons not to do so. All things being equal, the longer the track record of safety and effectiveness, the better.

Intention of Treatment

Treatment is given with four main benefits in mind:

1. to control or cure your disease, if possible,
2. to minimize your pain and distress,
3. to help you feel empowered, and
4. to help you feel hopeful.

When considering a treatment option, emphasize the first goal and give priority to effective science-based therapies. In most cases, doing so automatically helps you to meet the other three important goals of treatment in the long run, if not immediately. So, how do you choose a course of treatment?

Before you start comparing the relative value of two or more particular treatments, you need to know if you should be comparing them at all. You wouldn't compare a salmon filet with a candlestick if you were deciding what entree to serve your guests for dinner, even though both may be important elements of a romantic evening event. This may sound too obvious, but misunderstandings happen all the time when looking at treatments. You need to know what each treatment is intended to fix before you start to compare them.

For starters, divide treatments into "primary" and "supplemental." Primary treatments are aimed at the disease, the goal being to cure or control it. When talking about cancer, examples of primary treatments include radiation, chemotherapy, surgery, hormonal therapy, and immune therapies. So, for instance, you might compare the cure rates of chemotherapy alone versus surgery followed by chemotherapy. You would not compare chemotherapy against a nonspecific treatment intended to boost your appetite.

Types of Treatment According to Intention
- Primary treatment: a treatment aimed at your disease
- Supplemental treatment: a treatment to help the primary medical treatments work well or aimed at helping you obtain comfort or strength

In contrast, supplemental treatments are given in hopes of helping you obtain some physical or emotional comfort. Supplemental therapies may help you tolerate the primary treatments or help them work better. In the treatment of patients with cancer, pain medications, antibiotics, sleep aids, physical therapy, acupuncture, massage, meditation, prayer, and counseling are examples of supplemental treatments. These measures are important elements in your healing and may at times mean the difference in your outcome.

Judge the value of a treatment option in the context of the intention for which it is being prescribed. A treatment can be a wise choice when given with one intention, and not when given with another. For example, when biofeedback is prescribed in order to relieve your anxiety, it can be a good treatment choice. For purposes of treating a curable infection or malignancy, the same biofeedback is a poor treatment choice. Sometimes one treatment may have many possible benefits, and it is important to choose the treatment based on the main intention for which it is prescribed. After my doctor discussed my chemotherapy options for my fourth recurrence, he made his final recommendation, cheerfully concluding, "Wendy, this chemo regimen won't make you bald." Instead of feeling grateful, I was concerned. "Don't worry about if I'll be bald or not," I said. "Give me the chemo that gives me the best chance of getting well!" Of course, my oncologist had already determined that each of his final choices would give me an equal chance of getting better. He had focused on the hair-preserving benefit because, when all else is equal, that is a good reason to choose one over the other.

Keep the main goal of your treatment in mind when weighing options. Discuss with your physicians the treatments that are aimed at your disease, and choose from among them. Then, start the process all over again by considering treatments aimed at other problems such as nausea or fatigue, and choose from among these choices for these problems.

What is the intended goal of each of your treatments? How well does each of your options meet the four goals of treatment? Which option meets the first goal best?

Primary Treatment

When I was learning about my various primary-treatment options for my cancer, I found it helpful to put each option into one of three categories: conventional, investigational, or alternative.

Understanding Primary Treatments

	Conventional	*Investigational*	*Alternative*
Also called	standard; mainstream; regular	experimental	unconventional; complementary; unorthodox
Where used	American hospitals, clinics, and medical offices	clinical trials run in hospitals, clinics, and medical offices	outside mainstream medicine
Examples	surgery; chemotherapy; hormonal therapy; radiation therapy; immunotherapy	new drugs; old drugs being tested in as-yet unproven dosages, routes of administration, or combinations with other therapy	laetrile (apricot pit medicine); macrobiotics; homeopathy; herbs; nutritional supplements; laying on of hands

The value of these categories is that they distinguish the *strength of scientific knowledge* about each treatment's safety and effectiveness in particular medical settings, and thus your doctor's ability to evaluate the risks and benefits for you. This system helps you compare apples against apples when choosing your treatments, and to recognize when you are comparing apples against oranges. The features outlined in the table below will help you organize your choices and understand the advantages and disadvantages of each category of treatment.

Comparing Primary Treatments

	Conventional	*Investigational*	*Alternative*
Science based	√	√	
Subject to FDA oversight	√	√	
FDA approved	√		
Documented benefits against disease	√	*	
Favorable risk-benefit ratio in defined clinical situations	√		
Favorable risk-benefit ratio if prescribed for a patient	√	√	
Known risk profile	√	*	
Defined side-effect profile	√	*	* *

* Only in Phase III and IV trials and in population defined by Phase I and II trials
* * Only for some alternative therapies

Conventional Treatment

Conventional medicine is standard or mainstream medicine that is used widely in American hospitals, clinics, and doctors' offices. These treatments have evolved rapidly over the past thirty years, and all the newer therapies have been subjected to rigorous double-blind-placebo-controlled studies to determine their safety and efficacy. In contrast to alternative therapies, all conventional therapies have been studied in scientific settings and will continue to be as long as they are in use. Unlike investigational and alternative therapies, all conventional therapies have known risks, defined side-effect profiles, and documented benefits. Whether a treatment is designed in a high-tech research lab or plucked off an exotic plant, as long as its safety and efficacy have been demonstrated scientifically and validated with FDA approval, it can be used as conventional therapy.

Your personal physicians prescribe conventional therapies after ascertaining that the benefits outweigh the risks for you. Their judgment derives from

- knowledge of therapies that have been shown, based on scientific information and the judgment of the medical community, to have favorable risk-benefit ratios (i.e., the benefits outweigh the risks) when used in specific medical settings;
- knowledge of your unique medical situation.

For example, if you have a throat infection and are allergic to penicillin, your physician might prescribe erythromycin for you because the FDA has approved it for infections like yours in people who, like you, are allergic to penicillin. If, however, you are also allergic to erythromycin or suffering from profound nausea with your illness, your physician might prescribe yet another medication with a better benefit-to-risk ratio for you. Keep in mind that even when a conventional therapy doesn't offer you a cure, it often can delay the progression of your problem and improve your quality of life by minimizing medical complications such as pain, chemical imbalances, malnutrition, anxiety, and depression. As a Healthy Survivor, learn about conventional therapies that are available to treat or cure your disease.

Downsides of Conventional Treatments

Conventional therapies have downsides. For one, no conventional cancer therapy is guaranteed to work *in you* no matter how superb its track record. A conventional treatment that cures 98 percent of patients with your disease will fail to fix your problem if you fall in the 2 percent for whom the treatment doesn't work well. The uncertainty associated with conventional therapies is often seen as a big disadvantage of conventional therapies, especially if the chance of cure is low. It is not. No medical treatment on earth is a sure cure; the inability to guarantee a good response is a disadvantage shared by *all* medical therapies, conventional and otherwise.

> Uncertainty is a reality of every type of medical treatment, not just conventional therapies.

Given the uncertainty associated with illness and healing, the best you can do is to increase your chances of a good outcome as much as possible. This approach of stacking the odds of recovery in your favor is in keeping with the approach of going with your best odds in much of what you do. Imagine you want to unlock a cash box. Now imagine that you can choose between two keys, and the tag on one key reads "Opens 90 percent of boxes" while the tag on the other key says "Opens 10 percent of boxes." Which key would you try first? In the world of modern medicine, your physicians recommend treatments that have been demonstrated to offer people similar to you the greatest chance of cashing in on the treasure of good health.

Side effects and toxicities, both known and unexpected, are also seen as big disadvantages of conventional therapies. Like the uncertainty, these shortcomings are shared by every single intervention on earth. No treatment can be 100 percent guaranteed safe and nontoxic because the human body is infinitely complex and every person is unique. Some weird or unexpected reaction is always possible, even in response to placebos that contain no active ingredients.

How you perceive the risk of developing side effects makes a difference. Imagine a scenario where you are seriously ill and told that the best conventional therapy is very toxic and offers a 50 percent chance of cure. Understandably, you'd want a better option. This choice may feel as if you are voluntarily taking on the risks and discomforts of treatment, and, in return, getting only half a chance of cure. I suggest you look at it another way: Without treatment you have nearly a 100 percent chance of suffering or dying from your disease. Effective conventional treatments offer a solid chance of improving those odds to fifty-fifty. For patients with cancer or other serious diseases for whom no effective treatments are available, fifty-fifty sounds pretty good.

If you want to talk about the toxicity and risks of various treatments in a way that helps you make wise treatment decisions, discuss these risks in terms of your overall situation. Imagine a young child wandering onto a railroad track as a train approaches. If the parent calls to the child in a reassuring voice and gingerly pulls the child in hopes of making the experience less traumatic for the child, the parent's gentle and loving efforts may invite a disaster. Vigorously grabbing the child might break the child's arm and scare the bejeebers out of the kid in the process but with a good chance of saving the child's life. The parent can deal with the child's bruising and fright afterward. In a similar way, your physicians evaluate the risks of each of your treatment options in light of the total picture. They are looking at the risks of both your disease (the oncoming train) and your treatment (their attempt to improve or save your life). Keep in mind that whenever your physician prescribes a conventional treatment, it is always with the expectation that you will survive the treatment to benefit. Consequently, when talking about conventional therapies for serious illnesses, it is fine if you use a gentler therapy in hopes of sparing yourself the toxicities of rigorous conventional therapy *only if the gentler therapy also gives you as good a chance of controlling your disease.* For people with cancer, uncontrolled disease is the trump card when evaluating risks of cancer treatments. You must deal with the disease effectively, above all else.

Are you comparing the risks of treatment against the risk of suboptimally treated disease?

Hidden Risks

One risk that survivors often forget to include in the equation is the "unknown risk" associated with each type of treatment. This may seem a paradox: How can you evaluate the risk of something you can't know? Unknown risks can't be quantified. Even so, conventional therapies have fewer unknown risks than investigational and many alternative therapies.

Another hidden risk is the risk associated with delaying treatment. Sometimes patients, frightened by the prospect of side effects, take a long time deciding on a treatment. They feel safe because they assume that as long as they are not making a decision they are *suspending* their risk until they decide and begin treatment. The problem is that delaying treatment is the same as choosing "no treatment," an option that carries the risks of leaving your disease untreated or inadequately treated. As a Healthy Survivor, look at the risks of each treatment compared to the risks of the other treatments, and then compare these risks to those associated with leaving your disease untreated.

Perception of Increased Risk

Every action carries risk, not just the act of taking conventional therapies. When you recognize some of the reasons why conventional therapies can seem so risky and frightening compared to the normal risks you take, it may become easier to deal with the necessary risks of effective therapies. For example, whenever I've been scheduled to have a procedure or treatment, I've felt somewhat anxious while driving to the hospital. But I always focused on the impending medical procedures, not the trip, even though driving on Dallas's highways carries significant risk, too. The difference is that I'm used to hearing the daily radio reports about accidents and deciding that my mobility is worth the risk of driving. My decision has become so familiar and automatic that I don't think about it or feel the risk the same way I did the first time I drove. Yet, the first times I underwent chemotherapy and radiation therapy, I felt anxious because the risks were new and unfamiliar to me, and I had to think about them. With all the potential medical complications spelled out on consent forms, I was forced to acknowledge the risks and accept them with my signature before I could proceed with my treatments. I suspect that if I rarely rode in a car and then had to sign a detailed consent form before driving to the hospital, I'd feel different about the relative risks of cancer therapy and driving.

Practitioners of alternative therapies rarely ask patients to sign release forms that outline the risks of their treatments or the statistical likelihood of success. Certainly, when you buy an over-the-counter or mail-order treatment, you don't have to sign an informed-consent form. This omission encourages you to maintain an illusion of relative safety.

Another factor that may contribute to the sense of extraordinary risk from conventional medical therapies is that most people are not taking these same risks. Anytime you do something new to you and not done by the average person—skiing a high-level slope, skydiving, chemotherapy, organ transplantation—a stronger emotional response is triggered. As a Healthy Survivor, recognize when you are tempted to reject a conventional treatment option before giving it a fair shake against the other options.

Food and Drug Administration (FDA) Approval

Practitioners of conventional medicine use FDA-approved therapies to help heal patients. One bitterly disputed problem with FDA approval is the time lag between the discovery of promising new "evidence-based" treatments and their availability for use. The current method of proving a treatment to be scientifically sound requires a huge investment of time, not to mention the investment of money and people needed to develop, test, and approve a new treatment. Although this time lag is a real disadvantage that angers many patients who need and want answers today, this disadvantage is inextricably linked to the advantage *to you* of laborious scientific testing and critical evaluation by unbiased statisticians and scientists. When a treatment makes it through the FDA approval process, you can have confidence that it has been shown in rigorous tests to be effective with acceptable risks in the population studied.

The FDA has to balance the desire to minimize risk to individual patients (like you) with the desire to get effective treatments to people (like you) as soon as possible. When effective treatments take a long time to obtain approval, people are unhappy and say that the FDA is being too cautious. Then again, when approved treatments have to be recalled, people are unhappy and say that the FDA is not being cautious enough. Researchers and the FDA walk a fine line when deciding whether or not to approve a new drug; in general, they err on the side of safety.

Still, unexpected problems occasionally arise after a treatment is FDA approved and released for general use. In dramatic fashion, drugs have had to be recalled due to unanticipated toxicities not seen in the clinical trials in which they were initially tested. This is unavoidable because, when the risk is relatively low, problems become detectable only after millions of people use the intervention, far more patients than are ever involved in trials. Also, after therapies are released for general use, they are used by a wider variety of patients under less controlled conditions. For instance, unlike the typical patient in a trial who has been rigorously screened before treatment begins and who is followed closely during treatment, patients who use drugs after FDA approval

- may have co-existing medical conditions that increase their risks;
- may be taking additional therapies (e.g., for unrelated conditions) that increase their risks;
- may be monitored less closely.

At its most fundamental level, the mission of the Food and Drug Administration is to protect the public health. Yet, many Americans are skeptical of the FDA's ability to safeguard them, a distrust that has been fueled by the furor over approved drugs that subsequently proved to be dangerous for certain patients. For example, after the antidepressant drug Prozac was FDA approved, it was used widely and found to be associated with an increased risk of suicide in children and teens. So, years after the drug was approved, the FDA added a black-box warning to the prescribing information, signifying an extremely serious side effect of a prescription drug. In another example, the antiarthritis drug Vioxx was voluntarily taken off the market by the drug company because, after years of approved use, an increased risk of heart attack was brought to light.

Controversy revolves around how much the pharmaceutical companies and the FDA knew about these risks before and after the drugs received

FDA approval and about steps that might have been taken earlier to protect patients. Changes in financial arrangements have caused major shifts in who oversees safety, and how. Changes such as the new independent Drug Safety Oversight Board and the proposed "Drug Watch" Web page will help, but, clearly, problems exist with the FDA and drug companies.

What is a patient to do? While you are comparing treatments, you may be wondering what advantage FDA approval offers since it can't guarantee that a particular treatment is safe *for you*. Does FDA approval really matter at all? Yes, it does matter! When looking at any treatment that has made it through the FDA approval process, as explained above, you can have confidence that it has been shown in time-consuming, rigorous tests to be effective with acceptable risk in the population studied. Unlike alternative therapies that have not been scrutinized scientifically, treatments that have received FDA approval have been so examined. Sound information is available now that can enable your doctor to make a wise judgment about the benefits and risks to you. Information will continue to accrue as it is used more widely, and this additional information will help your doctors monitor and adjust your therapy.

FDA-approved therapies are often your best options.

The bottom line is that an FDA-approved treatment may be, and often is, the very best option for getting you better. Don't let safety and reporting concerns after a drug receives FDA approval keep you from the therapies that may help you most. To turn your back on conventional therapies is to throw the baby out with the bathwater. I am alive and my cancer is in remission thanks to conventional drugs discovered through research done at hospitals and pharmaceutical companies.

Although problems with drug safety will likely be around for quite a while even as policy improvements are made as a result of the Vioxx recall, you can take steps to minimize your personal risk of taking any FDA-approved therapies, as discussed in appendix V. You'll note that, in most cases, the following safeguards won't help you prevent problems caused by adding an alternative therapy to your medication regimen. Scientific information on the risks and benefits of doing so is not yet available.

Tips Before Beginning Any New Medication

- Talk with your health-care team to find accurate answers to specific questions, such as
  - What are the known risks of this drug, such as the risk of heart problems, kidney problems, nervous-system problems, depression, and so on?
  - Has this drug been used by patients who have the same conditions as you (your *other* medical conditions unrelated to the condition for which you are considering treatment)? If so, has the use of this treatment been associated with any increased risks?
  - Has this drug been used by patients who are also taking the same medication(s) as you are taking for other medical conditions? If so, has the use of this treatment been associated with any increased risks?
- Ask your pharmacist for information on the new drug and to check if it is safe to take with your other medications.
- If you want to find out more about the drug or your risk of taking it, see tips in Appendix IV.
- Let others be the guinea pigs. If a new drug for your condition comes on the market, don't be in a rush to use it unless you can't take any of the currently available therapies or they aren't working for you, or the new drug is clearly safer and/or more effective.

Thinking about the risks of medications may make you afraid to use *any* drugs unless they are *guaranteed* safe. Being wary is fine; in fact, it is good. Very good. But if you are expecting to use only totally risk-free treatments, you may deprive yourself of the benefits of drugs that can make you healthier and your life better. Remember: You may have to take risks to make your life better. An exaggerated concern about the risk of drugs could cause you to deprive yourself of healing therapies.

Tips While Taking Medication(s)

- Be alert to changes in your condition that may be related to your medication(s).
- Bring a written list of all your diagnoses and all your medications to every doctor visit.

- When you report a sign or symptom to your health-care team, remind them what medication(s) you are taking, no matter how infrequently and even if you've been taking it for years.
- Before any doctor prescribes an additional medication for any condition, review with him or her all your diagnoses and all your current medications.
- Before undergoing any procedure, no matter how minor and even if unrelated to the condition(s) for which you take medications, review with the doctor who is going to do the procedure (or who ordered the procedure) all your diagnoses and all your medications.

> If a new symptom or medical problem develops, ask your physicians, "Could this be related to my medications?"

A problem that begins soon after starting a new drug should make you think immediately about the new drug. But remember: Some adverse effects first appear months or years after starting a drug. So, whenever you develop a problem, make sure your physicians consider the possibility of your medications causing or exacerbating the problem. Get a second opinion, if necessary.

Off-Label Use of Conventional Therapy

Off-label use of drugs is very common. For example, a medication approved for one specific condition might be prescribed for a patient suffering from a similar, but different, condition. When Rituxan—the first monoclonal antibody therapy approved by the FDA for the treatment of cancer—became available, it was indicated for patients with a particular type of lymphoma. It is no secret that many cancer doctors prescribed it for patients with different types of lymphoma for which no satisfactory therapies existed. Why did they do this? Because their patients had diseases for which the best current therapies were disappointing, and, given the available scientific knowledge about the risks of the new drug, the potential benefits were felt to outweigh the risks. In many cases, this off-label use is supported by clinical studies, including randomized trials, and the only reason that the indication isn't formally added to the list of FDA-approved indications is a business one: The manufacturer has decided not to pursue it.

Another form of off-label prescribing occurs when a drug approved for use in a specific dose is prescribed in a different dose. Given what is known about the risks of the drug, the physician has weighed the potential benefits against the known risks and judged that it is a good treatment option for the patient. Ideally, if scientific studies are done, they will prove the safety and efficacy of using the drug in this way (a big "if" because the FDA rarely requires postapproval studies and pharmaceutical companies are not enthusiastic about subjecting their profitable drugs to these tests). You can still have confidence in off-label use of FDA-approved drugs, prescribed by an appropriate doctor, because their use is based on sound science with enough information available on the risks and benefits. And since you will be taking them in the context of conventional therapies, you will benefit from ongoing data that accrue.

FDA-approved, evidence-based treatments: the yardstick against which all other treatments are measured. Through sound scientific study, the benefits of these interventions have been shown to outweigh the risks in the tested population of patients.

FDA-approved, authority-based treatments: Based on their long history of success and use in the context of conventional and investigational medicine, the medical community has ascertained that the benefits outweigh the risks when used as prescribed. As these treatments are used in the context of conventional and investigational medicine, and as newer treatments become available, the risk-benefit ratio is fine-tuned.

FDA-approved, off-label treatments: These treatments have been FDA approved for use in one particular condition and are being prescribed for different conditions, or are being prescribed in different doses, via different routes, or in combination with other therapies. These treatments are based on scientific theory and what is known through scientific study about their risks. Your prescribing physician has ascertained that the potential benefits to you (unknown, but promising) outweigh the documented and potential risks.

The preceding table reviews the subcategories of conventional therapies. The purpose is not to confuse you but to give you some idea of the types of validation that exist for the various conventional treatments. In many cases, when you are exploring a specific conventional treatment, it is hard to find data from placebo-controlled trials of safety or effectiveness. That's okay because the crux of the issue is how all conventional therapies are similar: They are well-described treatments given in the context of science-based medicine and under constant scrutiny of your personal physicians who are looking for better answers to your medical problems.

Investigational Therapies

The next category of treatments given to cure or control your medical problem is *investigational* therapies. Also called experimental, these are treatments that are being evaluated by qualified scientists in research settings. When treatments look promising in studies performed in test tubes and on animals (preclinical trials), studies are developed that test these new treatments on people (clinical trials.) Preclinical and clinical trials provide useful and reliable information about treatments. When clinical trials prove a new therapy to be more effective, safer, or less toxic than current conventional approaches to a particular medical problem, the investigational treatment replaces it, becoming the new conventional way to treat that problem.

By definition, an investigational treatment *has not been proven better* than conventional therapies for treating the problem in question. Researchers may have some sense of what they expect from a treatment being studied but, until the studies are done and the results are analyzed, nobody knows if an investigational therapy is better or worse than conventional therapies. As an example, in the early and mid-1990s bone-marrow transplant for the treatment of metastatic breast cancer held promise both in theory and early studies. Many breast-cancer patients desperate for a better answer than conventional chemotherapy begged their doctors and insurance companies to approve bone-marrow transplants for them to be given *not* as part of a clinical trial. Why? They didn't want to take a chance that in a trial they would be relegated to the standard treatment arm of the study. They believed that transplant gave them the best chance and wanted it, even though the grueling treatment had never been proven more effective than standard chemotherapy. As it turns out, subsequent studies have not shown a survival benefit of transplant over conventional chemotherapy for most of these patients.

Clinical trials have two goals. The first has future patients in mind: to discover and explore therapies that work better than today's standard therapies in one way or another. New treatments may prove to be more effective, less dangerous, less expensive, easier to get, easier to administer, or have some other advantage. The researchers who act as your primary-care physicians while you are in the study have a moral obligation to allow you to participate in the trial only when it is ascertained that the risk-benefit ratio, based on everything that is known about the trial treatment and about you, is the best of your choices. And throughout the trial, they have an obligation to put your welfare above all else. Which brings me to the second, and most compelling, reason to consider receiving treatment in a trial: Treatment received in clinical trials may

A treatment available only in a clinical trial may be your best chance for improvement or cure.

prove to be better than any standard treatment. If you have an illness that is not curable or treatable with available standard therapies, an investigational treatment may represent your best chance for improvement.

Each time my cancer recurred, my physicians and I looked at standard treatment options and investigational therapies, balancing all the known and potential risks and benefits before making a decision. In 1993, none of the standard treatment options for my second recurrence offered me a chance for a lasting remission, and all were associated with significant toxicity. I decided to enter a trial for my type of cancer that was evaluating a promising agent—a monoclonal antibody that was part mouse and part human. Over the next four years, I entered three different trials of these monoclonal antibodies because each time the specific trial felt like the best balance of risks and benefits for me. Fortunately for me, the treatments worked as well as chemotherapy and without much toxicity. At the time, and in retrospect, the trial therapy was the best of all my choices in 1993, 1994, and 1997. By the time I needed treatment in 1998, the trial drug had been FDA approved as a standard therapy for my type of lymphoma, and I was able to receive it in my local oncologist's office. As it turns out, the investigational treatment I received in clinical trials has become one of the most commonly prescribed standard therapies for my particular type of lymphoma, improving life expectancy curves for the first time in decades.

Another benefit of participating in those trials was that they gave new meaning to my illness: I was helping researchers learn about treatments that might help other patients and future generations. Many trial subjects, even those whose disease marches on defiantly, take comfort and inspiration from the profound meaning given their illness through trial participation. That's all very heartwarming and romantic, but when making a treatment decision I advise you to look at trials from a purely self-interested point of view. The key question is: How might this cutting-edge therapy available only in a clinical trial help your medical condition? How do the risks and benefits of a trial therapy compare to those of your standard options? By obtaining sound knowledge about all your treatment options, you will have a sense of whether or not a clinical trial is a good option for you.

When you have a condition that is not reliably and easily corrected with conventional therapy, you should at least consider a clinical trial. Unfortunately, myth and misinformation surround trials. A common myth that frightens away potential patients with serious illnesses is the notion that if you enter a trial you might be denied effective treatment and, instead, be given a placebo. Rest assured, you would never be given "sugar water" when effective standard therapies are available. Rather, you would receive either the newer treatment or current standard therapy because these trials compare the investigational therapy against the best standard therapies. Recognizing the inherent risks in clinical trials, for the most part you can expect to do at least as well as you would with standard conventional therapies.

You may be concerned about the safety of the trial itself, knowing that some of the people in charge of decision-making about the trial have the trial—not the people being treated in the trial—as their foremost concern. As another line of defense in your favor, each and every research study using investigational treatments must be approved by a committee called an Institutional Review Board (IRB). The key responsibility of these boards is to make sure that the benefits of every research study are greater than the risks to each individual subject or patient who is enrolled in a trial at any phase of the trial. These boards report directly to the federal government, not to the institutions of which some of their members may be a part. For the past few years, I've been a patient advocate on a trial's safety monitoring board, a committee that monitors a trial's progress after IRB approval (and which is yet another line of defense for you). As a voting member, I've seen how this process works. Institutional Review Boards and safety monitoring boards are totally independent of pressures that might otherwise be placed on them by researchers. These layers of review are all designed to protect you, the patient.

As for being vulnerable to the rare researcher who has lost his or her moral compass and has ignored patients' rights or has made egregious and unforgivable errors, remember that someone like this is the exception. Institutional safeguards have been put in place at all levels of research to further decrease the potential for exploitation or malpractice. Fearing the rare bad apple may keep you from benefiting from the fruits of research. Clinical trials are not for everyone, and choosing to participate in a trial is a highly personal decision. Think through whether a clinical trial may give you your best chance at improvement.

Have you discussed with your doctors the option of entering a clinical trial?

Alternative Therapies

The third main category of treatment is alternative therapies, also called unconventional, unorthodox, or complementary. These are treatments designed and administered outside of mainstream (conventional and investigational) medicine and that are used *instead* of conventional or investigational therapy. By definition, *no alternative therapy has been scientifically proven safe and effective against serious diseases like cancer.*

Any "alternative therapy" that has been subjected to scientific study and proven at least as safe and effective as standard therapies is now considered a conventional therapy (or should be by any reputable doctor). Any alternative therapy that has been studied and proven ineffective should be lumped with quackery. Because this point is so important, I will repeat it: *No alternative therapy has been scientifically proven safe and effective in the treatment of cancer and other life-threatening diseases.*

Some alternative therapies do show promise in early scientific studies. But according to this classification system, a therapy that is being studied in clinical trials would be considered "investigational" when administered as part of a clinical trial and "alternative" when being administered outside of a clinical trial. So, for example, if high-dose vitamin C is administered to a patient with diabetes mellitus in one of the clinical trials being run by the National Institutes of Health (NIH), the therapy is "investigational"; whereas if the exact same therapy is given to a patient by a practitioner of alternative medicine, the therapy would be considered "alternative." Even though the drug itself may be the same, the circumstances are very different—the doctor will be monitoring in a scientific manner whether there is any effect on the health of the trial patients—so the risks for a patient with diabetes taking this vitamin C are different.

Make sure you have a clear understanding of the risks and downsides of using alternative therapies *instead* of conventional therapies for treating your disease. Since, by definition, no alternative therapies have been proven safe and effective in scientific study, you are not comparing apples against apples when comparing an unproven alternative therapy to a conventional therapy.

Confusion of Terms

All these terms—conventional, investigational, and alternative—are terribly confusing because people use a variety of terms for these three categories, such as "experimental" for "investigational" or "complementary" for "alternative." Some people use the word *complementary* for *supplemental*. In addition, CAM, the term adopted by the NIH, stands for complementary and alternative medical therapies, which lumps them together in many people's minds. Given the confusion of all these terms, it's not surprising that experts in these fields often disagree as to whether a specific treatment is conventional or alternative, and whether it is scientifically proven safe and effective.

As was illustrated a few examples earlier, the same treatment is called something different depending upon how it is used. For example, a vitamin preparation is "investigational" when administered as part of a clinical trial and "alternative" when taken outside of a trial, under the auspices of a practitioner of alternative medicine. Or, a specific drug may be conventional, but you may receive it in a different dose, via a different route, or in combination with other medications as part of a clinical trial, in which case the proper label for this otherwise standard treatment would be "investigational." An unconventional drug prescribed by an unconventional healer and taken instead of effective conventional therapy would be considered alternative. If taken along with conventional therapy, the same drug prescribed by the same healer would be considered complementary. What a mess.

Additional confusion arises because, in common usage, the word *alternative* means "option," "choice," or "another selection." Consequently, when doctors try to individualize your therapy so as to maximize the benefit and minimize the risk to you, they may talk about prescribing an "alternative" to the usual first-line therapy, meaning another choice of conventional treatment, and not an unconventional treatment. For example, both tetracycline and amoxicillin are conventional therapies, but your doctor may prescribe tetracycline as an "alternative" antibiotic to amoxicillin for your bronchitis. Tetracycline and amoxicillin might be called "two alternative therapies," meaning two selections of conventional therapies, and not meaning two out-of-the-mainstream therapies.

The Appeal of Alternative Therapies

You'd have to live on Mars to avoid hearing or reading about alternative therapies. Studies suggest that a majority of patients use some alternative therapies, often without informing their physicians. But scientific proof is lacking or has proven the therapy ineffective. What's going on here? To explore this question, let's look at how alternative therapies played into my survivorship. Before my cancer diagnosis, I understood, intellectually, the appeal of alternative approaches. When discussing alternative therapies with my patients, I tried to help them balance the risks and benefits of each treatment, conventional and otherwise, so that they could make the best decision for them. I saw my job as helping them to make *informed* decisions, not necessarily to follow my advice. I was both fascinated and dismayed by knowledgeable patients who pursued alternative therapies instead of effective conventional therapies.

When I became a patient, my understanding of the lure of alternative cancer therapies deepened. As explained in the prologue, I was only thirty-six years old and had three children under six when I was diagnosed with a type of cancer that the textbooks uniformly labeled "incurable." The first time I had cancer, I was bombarded with stories, information, and advice about diets and doctors, the mind-body connection, and alternative treatments for curing cancer. My knowing that no alternative therapy had been proven effective for treating cancer helped me file away the flood of articles, books, and audio- and videotapes that came my way, and dismiss the various theories of healing they presented. I renounced it all, but not without a twinge of hesitation. You see, while some people gently encouraged me to keep a more open mind, others' messages were more urgent: "Dr. Harpham, you must read about this treatment! It may save your life." A few tried to make me feel guilty, scolding my ignorance and stubbornness: "I can't believe you don't know about this cure."

And then there was my friend who was studying homeopathy. One could cast doubt on the motivations of suppliers of kooky concoctions. But she was a dear friend and only wanted me to get well. She truly believed she had a better answer for me than intravenous steroids and poisons; she thought I was making a mistake to reject homeopathy with its long history of a gentle, natural approach to curing all ills. On some level, to reject her suggestions was to snub her belief system. But I didn't believe in homeopathy, so I filed away her mailings, too.

That first year after my diagnosis, I was unwavering in my belief that conventional therapy gave me the best chance at survival, a faith that helped me accept the necessary discomforts and the risk of late effects of my chosen treatment, the so-called slash-burn-poison approach to cancer. Six months later, scan evidence of complete remission validated my faith in the science that saved me. At the same time, though, fear of recurrence and the passivity that characterize completion of treatment gave me my first real taste of the appeal of alternative therapies. Conventional medicine seemed impotent, poised only to react to the first signs of recurrence; alternative therapies tempted me with the promise of taking charge, of doing something to prevent my cancer from recurring. But I didn't investigate, still filing away the continuing trickle of articles and books on alternative therapies without really looking at them. My fear of recurrence was channeled, instead, into efforts at time-honored measures to enhance my recovery: eating well, resting, exercising, attending a support group and counseling, and prayer.

Two years later, after I'd been through aggressive chemotherapy and radiation therapy, my lymphoma recurred. Standard cancer therapies no longer offered me realistic hope of a lasting remission. I had to ask myself, "Am I still willing to bet my life on conventional medicine?" Sick and weak, scared and vulnerable, and painfully aware of what conventional therapies couldn't offer me, I opened my thick, dusty file on alternative therapies and began to read and talk about them with the mind of a scientist and the heart of a patient desperate to survive. "Let me look," I thought. After all, conventional medicine had missed the mark before, advising radiation for acne and infant formula over breast milk. I knew from my own training that our understanding of the roles of nutrition and spirituality in healing lag woefully behind our understanding of high-tech procedures and medicines. My memories of cancer-related leg pain and treatment-induced vomiting fed a rising fear of dying before my children were grown, and of leaving my husband a widower. If there was something, anything out there that offered me a better chance, I needed to know about it. "Let my doctors think me a fool," I thought, "If homeopathy, shark cartilage, or even snake oil can fix my cancer, I want it."

Tired of feeling sick and dreading feeling even sicker, I found the possibility that a gentle alternative therapy could cure me most seductive. Some alternative therapies offered me a sense of empowerment that I had not experienced when tethered to a radiation table or hooked up to an IV. Packaged pills and testimonials tugged at my hope while theories of antineoplasia, seemingly too simplistic or far-fetched before, now stoked my desire to control the disease that threatened my life. The lure of alternative therapies for curing cancer was powerful.

My dilemma clarified for me the contrast between conventional medicine and alternative therapies: Scientists are always skeptical—questioning "how" and "why," demanding proofs every step of the way. Conventional medicine is provisional and always will be. It represents the best treatments we have now with the expectation that better understanding and improved therapies will come along. In contrast, proponents of alternative therapies claim to possess an absolute truth about healing. While practitioners of conventional medicine don't make promises that can't be kept, alternative "healers" often do, asking patients to have faith in them, claiming to have the ultimate solution to their problem, often pointing to their long history of use, as if older or natural is always better. Sometimes older is better. A soup recipe handed down through generations or an oboist's age-old method of preparing a reed by hand may be hard to improve upon. But you won't catch me ironing my clothing with a heavy metal block like those used in colonial days or driving on tires that aren't radials. And I'd much rather have laparoscopic removal of my gall-

> Stack the odds for your recovery in your favor. Choose a primary therapy that gives *you* your best chance at improvement.

bladder and go home the same day with a Band-Aid dressing than undergo the old-fashioned major surgery that would require a lengthy hospital stay and leave me with a foot-long zipper scar.

Your illness is happening in your body. You have a right to choose what is best for you. Remember your goal when you look at any primary therapy, including alternative therapies aimed at treating your disease: to find the treatment that gives *you* your best chance at improvement.

Be sensitive to emotional issues that might be interfering with your ability to make what should be a rational decision (namely, choosing a course of treatment that stacks the odds in your favor). Especially when you don't have one clear "best" choice, these decisions are difficult. People are available to help you make wise decisions, such as your doctors and nurses, social workers and psychologists, chaplains, and friends and family. Ultimately, you decide what role, if any, alternative therapies have in your survivorship. This decision depends on your condition, what conventional medicine has to offer you, and the specific alternative therapy you are considering. Only you can know the best choice for you. What matters is that you obtain sound knowledge, so that you make informed decisions and never look back saying "I wish I'd known then what I know now."

What role, if any, are alternative therapies playing in your survivorship? How often do people encourage you to try alternative therapies?

Supplemental Therapies

As part of your treatment plan, your specialist may prescribe supplemental therapies such as antinausea medications, hormones, acupuncture, biofeedback, or meditation to calm anxiety, and massage to relax muscles. These treatments are prescribed to help your treatments work well, or to help you stay as healthy, comfortable, and hopeful as possible. You benefit when you invest the effort to learn about your options in supplemental therapy. Be forewarned: Finding reliable scientific information about supplemental therapies may be even harder than finding out about primary treatments. If your specialists are busy diagnosing and treating you with conventional therapies, they may seem to have too little time, interest, or knowledge about various supplemental therapies such as nutrition or exercise. If so, you'll have to obtain sound knowledge about supplemental therapies from other reliable sources like your nurses and allied health professionals.

Nutritional, Herbal, and Vitamin Supplements

Nutritional or dietary supplements deserve special mention because they are so widely available and can be obtained without a prescription. Since the Dietary Supplement Health and Education Act of 1994 (DSHEA) was passed, supplements are, with some exceptions, any product intended for ingestion as a supplement to the diet. This includes vitamins, minerals, herbs, botanicals, and other plant-derived substances, and amino acids (the individual building blocks of protein) and concentrates, metabolites, and constituents and extracts of these substances.

Nutritional supplements that are proven safe and effective in scientific studies may be prescribed as a conventional medicine. For example, physicians prescribe the vitamin folic acid to pregnant women to help prevent neural tube defects and calcium pills to patients with osteoporosis. However, when dietary supplements are used outside of conventional medicine and their safety and effectiveness for a particular condition have not been proven scientifically, these supplements become a form of alternative therapy.

Manufacturers do not have to provide information to the FDA to get a dietary supplement on the market. Since you can buy them off grocery shelves without a prescription, they may seem to be as safe as apples. Nothing could be farther from the truth. Supplements do not have to prove safety or effectiveness even though they contain chemicals that can affect your body. Ironically, it is the chemicals they contain that give them their claims to healing, yet they are considered "natural" and "nonchemical" therapies.

At best, scientific information is available on the risks of a particular dietary supplement, but these potential problems are rarely noted on the packaging. Unlike drugs and medical devices, nutritional supplements are exempt from FDA regulations that demand that the packaging outline the risks of taking the product. And it is legal to sell a supplement that is not exactly what it says it is or that doesn't do exactly what it promises to do. Well-done studies have shown that different bottles of supplements often supply variable amounts of the supposedly active ingredient. Sometimes pills and liquids contain little or none of the reputedly active ingredient! No matter how much you learn about a dietary supplement, if it is possible that you are not getting what you think you're getting, you could be in trouble. In addition, supplements are rarely tested in combination with conventional therapies such as antibiotics, heart medicines, or chemotherapy. Nor are they packaged with warnings about drug interactions even though supplements may cause serious problems when you take them in conjunction with your conventional medications.

Regard the claims of nutritional supplements with the same skepticism as you regard anecdotes. The information in ads may or may not be true, and can't tell you anything about how the treatment might help *you*. Only when a supplement has been proven safe and effective in scientific studies, and when a respected company that is accountable manufactures it, can you use the supplement with the same confidence you use FDA-approved drugs. Make sure you tell your doctors of any supplements you are taking. They need to know because the supplement may interfere with other of your medications. If you are using a supplement with the approval of your treating physician, make sure you buy products manufactured by a reputable pharmaceutical company.

Have you discussed supplemental therapies with your physicians?

Choosing Supplemental Therapies

When evaluating supplemental therapies, repeat the process you used when evaluating your primary treatment options. Assess the source of information and the strength of the data available on the treatment. The stakes may not be as high as when choosing a primary treatment for your underlying disease, but an attitude of caveat emptor—let the buyer beware—still applies. If you end up choosing a harmless but ineffective supportive treatment, all you lose is some time, energy, and money. But some supplemental therapies can affect your quality of life dramatically, for good or bad and can, on occasion, threaten your health or life. As a Healthy Survivor, choose supplemental therapies with the same care as your primary therapies, and keep your physicians informed.

Deciding on a Course of Treatment

Now that you've obtained sound information about your primary treatment options and your options regarding supplemental therapies, how
do you decide on a course of treatment? The bad news is that you can't
know for sure if any treatment is going to work for you until you try it.
The good news is that you can stack the odds in your favor as well as possible. Physicians practicing conventional medicine help you gauge your
odds of getting better and your odds of having problems related to the
therapy. Use statistics as your starting point, so you can know which
treatments give you the best chance of improvement or cure.

Over the years, many people have applauded my decision to enter a
clinical trial in 1993. To them, I obviously made a wise decision because
I'm doing well now. If, however, the trial drug hadn't worked for me, I
wouldn't look so smart. Or, if I'd had a terrible reaction to the experimental drug and I'd died, many observers would have concluded that I'd
made a bad decision. Some might even generalize that patients should
never agree to participate in clinical trials.

Actually, no matter what had happened to me medically, it was the
wisest choice for me at that time. I'm just grateful
that my wisest choice turned out to be a treatment
that worked well. Since factors beyond patients'
control also affect their outcome, many other
patients make equally wise choices but aren't as
fortunate. When you are a patient, the most you
can do at any decision-making juncture is to make
a wise choice that stacks the odds in your favor.

> The most you can do at any decision-making juncture is make a wise choice.

Hopefully, the treatment will get you well. If it does, celebrate. If not, start
again, giving every effort to making wise decisions based on where you
are now.

Realistic Options

When I had my second recurrence, my oncologist outlined all my treatment options. I didn't like any of them! I wished I had a better option.

But, accepting the limits of my realistic choices and focusing on them allowed me to work with my physicians to make a wise treatment decision and move forward. Wishing for something you can't have can hurt you. The classic scenario is the young attractive woman who can't seem to find a suitable mate. She immediately compares every eligible bachelor to her imaginary ideal beau and dismisses him as "too this" or "too that" before any real relationship has a chance to develop. In a similar way, patients who keep looking for a better treatment, rejecting therapies that seem to offer less, may sacrifice the realistic options that can help most. This feeling of wanting an ideal treatment can be subconscious, with a lingering sense that you're missing something better, or that

> When evaluating the risks you might have to take, remember: Your illness or injury changes the equation.

you are getting a raw deal if you proceed with wisely chosen (but costly, in some way) treatment.

What helped me most when treatment was rough was this: Illness changed the equation. I would never agree to take chemotherapy or radiation therapy if I were well. But I wasn't well. Given my illness, the benefits of these toxic treatments made them desirable options. Regarding risks you are willing to take, your illness or injury changes the equation. In general, when facing a serious or life-threatening condition, most patients are willing to try treatments that are riskier, more unpleasant, and more expensive than when dealing with a relatively minor problem. Your decisions are very personal. Look at your treatment choices as objectively as possible and choose from among those that offer real hope.

Decision Tools

Once you've obtained sound knowledge about each of your treatment options, how do you narrow down your choices and make a wise treatment decision? I suggest you find a tool that compares your options and, in as rational a manner as possible, helps you match those treatments that best meet your personal goals and needs. Work with your physicians to summarize what you've learned about each treatment choice and to compare and contrast them before making your decision. Each treatment option may entail accepting some level of discomfort, expense, and uncertainty. Your job is to figure out the most acceptable balance of risks and benefits, or disadvantages and advantages, in light of your personal needs, values, and beliefs. Bring the best of what you know to the decision. Embrace the hope offered by your treatment.

One way to manage the information is to answer the questions presented below for each of your treatment options. Not only will doing so clarify and simplify what is known about each of your choices; it will also highlight what is not known. Many times the answer to a question will be "Nobody knows." Personalize your list of questions by including factors that are important to you such as "Will it interfere with my fertility?" or "Is this treatment available close to home?" Obviously, each question does not carry equal weight. Again, how you prioritize the importance of each question is a personal issue.

Questions for Weighing Treatment Options

- What is the remission rate of this therapy for my condition?
- What is the cure rate of this therapy for my condition?
- What is the chance for improvement?
- What are the short-term risks of the treatment?
- What is the risk of dying from this treatment?
- What are the potential side effects and complications?
- What are the long-term risks?
- Will taking this treatment now limit my use of other treatment options in the future?
- What are the costs of treatment?
- Where is the treatment given?
- Who prescribes or administers the treatment?

HARPHAM'S DECISION TOOL

Another approach is to use the Harpham Decision Tool. You may find it especially helpful when you don't like any of your options. This tool is a model, and the categories and ratings are just suggestions. You can use it exactly as described, or modify it to suit your personal situation, values, or risk-taking preferences. In the grid below, fill in each of the boxes with a rating:

+ + + + = **very big advantage**   - - - - = **very big disadvantage**

+ + + = **big advantage**   - - - = **big disadvantage**

+ + = **advantage**   - - = **disadvantage**

+ = **slight advantage**   - = **slight disadvantage**

0 = **neutral**   ? = **information not available**   Rx = **treatment**

	Standard Option #1	*Standard Option #2*	*Investig. Option #1*	*Investig. Option #2*	*No Rx*
Remission rate (disease undetectable after Rx)					
Duration of remission					
Response rate (disease improved after Rx)					
Cure rate					
Short-term risks of Rx (infection, heart disease, bleeding, death, etc.)					
Long-term risks of Rx (second cancers, heart disease, osteoporosis, etc.)					
Limits other Rx options (other options too risky or less effective after Rx)					
Length of Rx course					
Effect of Rx on work/home					
Your costs (medications, travel, child care, etc.)					

This decision-making tool helps you choose the best treatment for you based on the most accurate and up-to-date information available to you today. When done, you'll see a lot of pluses and minuses, and possibly some question marks in the grid. The number and pattern of pluses and minuses can help you rank your treatment options from best to worst. You may have to base your final treatment decision on incomplete information because new treatments won't have available information on long-term risks and benefits until years from now, when enough time has transpired since these treatments came into use.

Ratings must be based on accurate information from reliable sources such as your specialists, the medical literature, and reputable disease-specific organizations. For purposes of this decision-making tool, ratings must not be based on anecdotal stories, your intuition, or your sense of hope about each treatment. Be sure to review your table with your physicians. Other people might be able to help you, too, such as your family doctor, other survivors who have been through these treatments, and a counselor. Don't worry about getting the ratings exact. As you use a pencil to fill in all the boxes, you can adjust entries you filled in earlier.

Temporary side effects are not included in the grid because when choosing a course of therapy, it is assumed that you are willing to deal with temporary treatment-related side effects and discomforts that are not health or life threatening. When you narrow your options down to two or three equally good ones, then you can look at temporary side effects as important factors that can help you choose one good option over another.

Make a decision based on the grid and then wait, if you have time. When I've had a couple of equally good choices (or equally frightening ones, as the case may be), one trick I've used is to imagine that I've decided on the first option, and see how I feel about it. Then, a day or two later, I switch and imagine I've decided on the second option, and see if I feel better or worse about my decision. Playing this mind game helps me get a feeling about the wisest route for me.

As long as waiting a short while is safe, take the time needed to make your decision. For many people, myself included, making the final decision is the hardest phase of survivorship. If you find yourself wanting to pick a treatment just to be done with the stress of deciding, remember that a wise decision will minimize your distress in the long run. It is worth the wait. Then, as soon as your decision is made, you will be able to let go of much of the distress that accompanies looking at all the possible problems and risks. You'll be able to focus on helping the treatments work well and nourishing hope that you will have a good outcome.

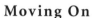

Who is helping you make wise treatment decisions? What tools are you using?

Moving On

Healthy Survivorship depends on more than just knowing the medical facts and choosing the best medical treatments. You need to understand what is happening to you—the real, whole "you"—when your body is sick or injured, and what you can do to make things better in all spheres of your life. Only by obtaining knowledge about the effects of illness or injury on your emotions can you respond to changes and challenges in life-enhancing ways. The next chapter will discuss making your life better by obtaining knowledge about your emotions.

Using Your Emotions

A few weeks earlier, my scans had confirmed what we'd all hoped: Six cycles of intensive chemotherapy had melted my lymphoma like water splashed on the Wicked Witch of Oz. My family had weathered the storm of my treatment. With my cancer in remission, our life could get back to normal. So why was I feeling anxious and unhappy? Why, now, were things unraveling at home?

Knowledge about Emotions

If you have a lump in your groin, the presence of the lump is a fact. All facts—pieces of information about the world—are objective, without feelings, hopes, or agendas attached to them. But once you feel the lump and realize something is wrong, the *fact* of your lump becomes something different. Now your emotions are stirred, and these emotions give the lump *meaning*. It is through your senses *and* your emotions that you experience the world around you. After discovering the lump, your efforts to obtain and process objective information about it can be mired in emotions, even when you believe that remaining dispassionate is in your best interests. Your reactions and outlook while dealing with the lump shape your important relationships and quality of life.

Whatever is happening in your life, emotions will shape your perception of and response to serious illness. You will find that obtaining knowledge about the medical aspects of your illness, alone, is not enough. You also need to learn about the interplay between your illness and your emotions. In the context of survivorship, talking about knowledge and emotions is like discussing the chicken and the egg. Your emotional state affects what you learn, and what you learn affects your emotions, which affect how much you learn! So what should you study first: the medicine of your illness or the emotions of it? My answer is that Healthy Survivorship is an ongoing learning process, and you'll probably go back and forth. Whether you learn about emotions before, simultaneously with, or after learning some of the medicine of your illness, understanding the emotions that accompany illness will help you use them in ways that help you to get good care and to live fully.

Strong Emotions

While trembling in my patient's gown, I learned that a diagnosis of serious illness is as much an emotional as a physical problem for the patient. After I got home from the hospital and the news began to sink in, my emotions were more powerful and disturbing than any I'd ever experienced. Being a patient, in pain, unable to work, and dependent were all new and alienating circumstances. The totally unfamiliar, unsettling intensity of my emotions made my situation all the more distressing, causing me to ask, "Why can't I handle this better? Am I weak? Have I gone nuts?"

The patient in me needed to be reminded of what the doctor in me already knew: Powerful emotions are a normal part of a serious diagnosis, and I was reacting appropriately. My fear, sadness, and sense of disorientation would calm down after a while. My grit and competitiveness would get me through. You can expect strong emotions at the time of diagnosis, if complications or setbacks occur, and during transitions (even good transitions such as when you first go home from the hospital or when you complete your treatments). Expecting intense emotions doesn't make them go away any faster, but it eliminates the additional stress of worrying about them, or trying to fight or hide them. Accepting your emotions makes it easier to use them all—the positive *and* negative emotions—to your advantage.

What strong emotions did you feel when first diagnosed or when a complication or setback occurred? What strong emotions have you been feeling recently?

Paying the Toll

The logic behind the first step to Healthy Survivorship—obtaining knowledge—is clear: Knowledge is power. But, as you already know if you have ever had a tense discussion about a problem with a loved one, bringing the cold facts out into the open can be highly emotional. Even for deeply committed couples, it takes courage and tact to discuss upsetting topics that affect them deeply. Only the rare person can keep a perfectly open mind and listen calmly.

Like the coins you toss into a highway toll basket, the time, energy, and emotional strain of obtaining knowledge about your illness and its ramifications are the costs of opportunities. I believe the costs are worth it because learning the truth earns you the chance to choose your best route to healing. And you don't get off scot-free if you choose not to obtain knowledge. Let's say you develop a backache that is slowly getting worse. It takes a lot of energy to reassure yourself ("It's nothing") when the rational part of you knows that your symptom *might*, indeed, signal a problem. If loved ones are worried about your pain, you also have to deal with *their* fear and frustration. The longer you wait, the more negative emotions will have piled up when you do, finally, find out what's wrong with your back. The expense of not obtaining knowledge applies if your problem is an emotional conflict, too, because it takes a lot of energy to live with ongoing tensions. When you pay the toll and learn about what is happening in your life, you are controlling your emotions and not letting your emotions control you.

Wouldn't every patient who wants to get better learn the essential information needed to get better? Wouldn't they do the right things to get better no matter what they are feeling? In a word, no. Fear, sadness, confusion, helplessness, anger, loss of self-esteem, jealousy, resentment, embarrassment, disappointment, and anxiety can form a complex web of unpleasant emotions that becomes an obstacle to Healthy Survivorship for even the most well-intentioned and well-motivated patient.

What thoughts and actions help you pay the toll?

Signals and Reactions

A tidbit that helps me through the rough times of my survivorship is this: Unpleasant emotions are not the problem but the body's way of announcing or responding to a problem. Knowing this, whenever I feel upset, angry, or confused, I sit down and try to determine, "Are these uncomfortable feelings the *signal* of a problem or the *reaction* to a problem?" Despite my analytic skills as a clinician, every now and then I need to talk with a friend, my husband, or the hospital social worker to sort out the underlying cause of my distressing feelings. Just as I can't look in my own ear to diagnose an earache, I can't always see behind my own emotions.

Unpleasant emotions are the body's way of announcing or responding to a problem.

It is not as important what your emotions *are* as what you *do* with them. The first step toward using your unpleasant emotions toward healing is to determine whether they are the signal of or the reaction to a problem. Here's an example: While recovering from my second course of treatment, the universal greeting "How are you?" irritated me, causing me to avoid certain people for fear of being asked. I recognized my edginess and anger as a signal of a problem. What my problem was I had no idea! So I called my good friend Debbie and spilled out my frustration. "Deb, they don't say, 'How are you?' but 'How *ARE* you?'" Debbie said that they didn't mean anything by it and I was being oversensitive. I didn't agree. Someone would ask, "How are you, Wendy?" and I'd answer, "Fine," and they'd double-check with raised eyebrows and chin tilted ever so slightly, "Really?" or "Are you still in remission?" It was not my imagination. People weren't simply saying "Hi," they were asking for my latest scan results.

Talking with Debbie and writing in my journal helped bring underlying tensions to the surface, such as how I had to absorb the disappointment and fear that splintered others' words of comfort. And how, if I happened to be enjoying a moment of forgetting about cancer, the concerned look behind "How are you?" snapped me back into being a cancer patient against my wishes. At the heart of my distress, being asked "How are you?" rattled my heightened sense of vulnerability by virtue of its literal meaning—"How am I?"—and my sense of "I don't know! I'll find out when I have my checkup."

These and other insights helped me understand the source of my emotional distress: I was having trouble dealing with my sense of vulnerability and the uncertainty about my future. Now that I understood why I was bothered, further talking and writing led me to healthy ways of dealing with them. *Using* my uncomfortable emotions encouraged my healing. Ever since my discussions with Debbie, "How are you?" no longer triggers even a twinge of discomfort. In fact, I like and appreciate when people ask, taking their question as a sign of their concern and love for me.

Tips for Dealing with Unpleasant Emotions
- Determine *what* you are feeling (e.g., sadness, anger, frustration).
- Determine *the source* of your feeling (i.e., why you are feeling the way you are).
- Determine if your feelings are lifting you up or pulling you down.
- Determine if your feelings are helping you get good care and live fully.
- Find ways to transform negative emotions into healing forces.
- Find ways to let go of emotions that are only hurting you.

If you feel a strong negative emotion, you don't have to sit down and start analyzing your every conversation and action. Uncomfortable feelings that are fleeting can be let go, without ever understanding or doing anything about them. However, pay attention to unpleasant emotions that persist or recur time and again, or that keep you from doing something you need to do to get better.

Are your emotions the signal of or reaction to a problem? Who can help you sort out the underlying cause of your emotions?

Feeling-ectomy

When unpleasant emotions are not *the signal* of a problem, they are often *the reaction* to a problem. You may be furious about a delayed diagnosis, sad over your loss of independence, or frustrated with miscommunications with your doctor's scheduling clerk. During the months after closing my medical practice, it was no mystery to anyone why I immediately got weepy whenever reminded of my office. In situations like these, you know exactly what problem is triggering your emotional reaction.

What do you do with your emotional reactions? A variety of factors may push you to ignore or suppress your strong negative emotions. Appearances, for one. Handling a crisis "well" in our society implies handling the problem calmly. But for Healthy Survivors, handling a situation well means handling it in whatever way helps you to get good care, adjust, and move forward.

> Handling a situation well means handling it in whatever way helps you to get good care, adjust, and move forward.

Why in the world should you feel perfectly calm when you first learn that you have a new medical problem? At the very least, your routine is disrupted as you anticipate undergoing treatment that will be uncomfortable and inconvenient. Feeling fear, anger, and other negative emotions shows that you understand what is going on (a good thing!). Expressing your negative feelings creates opportunities to *use these emotions* to heal. I know that the news of my recurrent cancer ignited fear but also stoked my maternal fires, energizing me with courage and determination in preparation for challenging times.

Another reason people may try to suppress ugly emotions is that these feelings are uncomfortable. When going through a particularly rough spot in my survivorship journey, I joked about wanting a "feeling-ectomy" because my negative emotions were making me miserable. I walked around, repeating in my head a line from one of Tina Turner's songs, "I don't want to hurt no more!" The problem was that to fight or hide my unpleasant emotions would be to deny myself their healing powers. And, a feeling-ectomy would sacrifice all the positive feelings that could help me get well and that make life worth living—feelings of courage, excitement, curiosity, joy, pride, and love. No, I don't want to avoid my emotions; as a Healthy Survivor I want to embrace them, painful as some of them may be, to help me heal and live fully.

You may be someone whose nature is to bob and weave through life, unable to relate to those of us who feel battered by life's ups and downs. Lucky you! Nothing wrong with that. You are doing fine, taking everything in stride and not worrying about anything *as long as you understand what is going on and your composure is sincere.* I admire people who are easygoing and confident of a good outcome in tough situations. Then again, I am envious of people who are tall and multilingual, or good with plants. But the fact is that I am *not* like that (not naturally, anyway). So while other newly diagnosed cancer patients are Healthy Survivors by sailing smoothly as if on a calm lake, I was a Healthy Survivor after my diagnosis by riding the ocean waves of my initial fear and sadness.

Believe me, if tears cured cancer, I would never have needed chemotherapy. Prompted by my losses and the stress of my treatment, I cried and cried for months until I got through my grief and fear. Please don't think you are supposed to cry or you *must* cry after getting bad news. But if you feel the urge to cry, and if it is hard to stop crying, then go ahead and cry. At least you will feel better, and you won't be wasting precious energy stifling your true feelings. At best, crying may have healing powers of its own, healing your emotions if not your body.

Fear, anger, and confusion fade with the passage of time and the benefit of sharing. Courage and love of life can flourish. You can learn and grow today in ways that help you tomorrow. Although it was painful and sometimes embarrassing, expressing my emotions during my first round of chemotherapy helped me get through—and become stronger. When I faced later recurrences, I didn't need to cry and I didn't feel as afraid. Now, whenever problems arise that stir unpleasant emotions, I seek out ways to *get through* my feelings (not to get around them) as soon as possible. Like a power nap, my "power-venting sessions" have helped me accept and adjust to unwanted changes and direct my attention toward solutions and happiness as quickly as possible. I like to think of it this way: Medical treatment makes me feel lousy physically while helping me get better, and expressing my unpleasant emotions makes me feel lousy emotionally while helping me heal.

Should your disease be incurable or untreatable with current therapies, allowing your feelings to surface enables you to use your positive and negative emotions to help you move through the various stages of grief and acceptance, and to embrace the life you still have. If your emotions are overwhelming or counterproductive, get professional help. You may never have needed counseling before. In the setting of illness, assessing your own emotional state can be like checking the back of your head: You need a mirror to see it. Professionals are trained to help you understand and use your emotions toward Healthy Survivorship, and professionals are more objective than family and friends. Even for psychological or social troubles I could have worked through on my own, obtaining professional assistance helped me get to a good place faster. More important, counseling helped me foster my positive emotions and grow as a person, much more so than had I worked my way through my emotions on my own.

With whom can you share your emotions? What do you think about professional counseling?

Using Your Emotions to Heal

Your emotions affect how you feel physically. The summer I underwent radiation to my neck and upper chest, I expected it would be totally painless, like having a Polaroid picture taken, and that seven to fourteen days later I might notice skin burn, dry mouth, and trouble swallowing. The first day of radiation to my neck and upper chest, I was lying strapped onto the table, holding still, unable to swallow because my neck was fixed in a hyperextended position by a plastic mask. The technicians left the room, and the light went on accompanied by the buzz of the machine. After thirty seconds, my skin got warm, which surprised me. But my skin was definitely warm and getting warmer. After the treatment was completed, I told my doctor about my skin heating up. Matter-of-factly, he said I'd imagined the sensation because I was scared.

Someone else might have been offended by his flip response, but I took it as a useful piece of information and was relieved because the thought had crossed my mind that they had accidentally given me too much radiation. Mixed in with my relief was a new concern: Am I crazy? (Is my doctor crazy?) I imagined that? No way! As I tried to explain to myself how the vivid sensation could have all been in my mind, I remembered long-forgotten events such as air-raid drills in elementary school, and all my attempts to avoid exposure to radiation at the dentist's office and while working with radioactive tracers during my tenure in neurobiology research. I concluded that I had a long-standing fear of radiation that expressed itself in physical symptoms even though the high-dose radiation was my choice.

The next day, I lay still as they strapped me into my mask, wondering what I would feel. What did I feel? Nothing. Absolutely nothing. Amazed that my fear could generate a powerful experience of physical warmth that was only in my mind, I appreciated the power of my emotions to help me heal. I consciously redirected my knowledge of the power of radiation to my advantage, visualizing the strong radiation easily killing all my cancer cells. Did it help my cancer go away? Maybe, but I wouldn't bet the family farm on it. Did it comfort me? Definitely. Did it hurt me in any way? Absolutely not.

When possible, transform negative emotions into positive ones. If this is impossible with some of your feelings, find ways to suppress or let go of harmful emotions. Just as important, nurture your life-affirming emotions. Your sense of confidence that you can tolerate therapy can help you experience hunger after therapy, and your sense of hope that you are getting better can diminish your experience of physical pain. I cannot emphasize enough that what matters most is what you do with your emotions, not what emotions you experience.

Tips on Emotions and Illness

- Emotions are a defining part of being human.
- Some of your emotions can prevent you from getting good care or living fully.
- Most of your emotions—negative and positive—can be used in ways that help you.
- You can learn to redirect or let go of emotions that are hurting you.
- Emotions are more manageable when shared with people who understand and care.

Right now, are your emotions helping you get good care? Are they helping you live fully?

Fear

Where do all these intense emotions come from? One of the chief fuels for intense emotions is fear, the emotional discomfort caused by awareness of imminent danger. When the diagnosis is serious, fear of death is a major emotion accompanying a new diagnosis, even if death is not a likely scenario in the near or foreseeable future. Other fears compound the intensity of fear: fear of pain, fear of treatment, fear of changes in body function and appearance, fear of abandonment by family, friends, co-workers, or the health-care team itself, fear of poverty, fear of the future, fear of loss, and fear of the unknown. From the time of diagnosis on, fear may try to be your ever-present companion.

Fear is not all bad. Fear of heights when you are walking too close to the edge of a canyon and fear of heart disease when you are trying to stop smoking are good fears to have. From an evolutionary point of view, these fears confer a survival benefit, pushing you to do the right thing to protect your life. In contrast, panic or undirected fear that accompanies a new diagnosis or medical setback is debilitating. Fear becomes troublesome when it keeps you from reporting a worrisome symptom or pursuing an effective therapy. In order to become a Healthy Survivor, especially during the first weeks after a diagnosis, learn to appreciate helpful fears and tame counterproductive fears.

> Learn to appreciate helpful fears and tame counterproductive ones.

How? Acknowledge them. Which fears are like a child's under-the-bed ogres imagined in the dark of night? Shine the light of knowledge on them and see these fears disappear. Maybe you fear your treatments. Even if the going is rough, it helps to know that millions of ordinary people have tolerated similar treatments and now enjoy good health. In an almost-magical way, giving voice to your fears—writing them down on paper or describing them to someone who cares—can make the object of your fear less formidable, even when nothing objective has changed about your situation.

You may benefit, too, from taking life in bits, rather than thinking about and trying to absorb the next few months or years all at once. Separate out and deal with only the fears that are affecting you now. When you are about to have surgery, you don't need to be worrying about the bills that will be arriving in a few weeks. When you are newly diagnosed, don't worry about recurrence or other longer-term concerns. You can and will deal with them later.

List destructive fears that need to be addressed now, and divide them into ones that you can do something about and those that you cannot. For the former, outline how you will tackle them. For example, if your immune system is compromised and you are afraid of becoming infected, use your fear to motivate you to find out how to minimize your risk of infection. Or, if you've just completed treatment, and you feel almost paralyzed by fear of getting sick again, learn how to (1) optimize your health through diet, exercise, medications, and whatever else applies to your situation; (2) detect problems early; and (3) use remaining fear in

life-enhancing ways or let go of the fear that remains. When facing illness, fear may be unavoidable but it is manageable and can be channeled
in healing ways.

Situations that elicit fear are tests of faith. As will be discussed in chapter 10, the fear as well as the anger and confusion surrounding your illness can become opportunities to clarify your spiritual beliefs. You may
rededicate your faith or find faith for the first time, or you may find out
or reinforce the fact that you do not believe in God. Which of these is the
surest path to Healthy Survivorship depends on which belief system
helps you in life-affirming ways. Knowing what you believe—whatever
that may be—can help you focus on the task at hand and feel at peace.

Don't assume that deep spiritual faith eliminates all fear. I've been
more accepting of my fear since hearing the story of a spiritual guide
whose peaceful wisdom comforted thousands at their deathbeds, yet
when he got sick, he cried out, "I'm scared! I don't want to die!" Human
beings are hardwired to feel fear when threatened. Don't assume that if
you feel fear you have weak faith. I venture that for most people, spiritual
faith doesn't prevent fear; it helps you live in harmony with your fear.

*What are your fears? What techniques help you
tame these fears?*

The Deep, Dark Well

A young boy passes an old well every day on his way to school. Fear keeps
him from walking near it or peering over the edge like the kids who enjoy
listening for the delayed clink of dropped pennies. From the time he
leaves home until the moment he enters his school building, his fearful
heart beats fast and he can't think about anything but the deep, dark well.
One day his best friend takes him by the hand, leads him to the well, and
encourages him to take a look. The boy's head swirls with a wave of nausea until his eyes gradually adjust to the dark and he can make out the

bricks lining the uppermost few feet of the well. The longer he looks, the steadier and less afraid he feels. Slowly, he inches his gaze down the bricks, lower and lower until the bricks fade into the darkness. Forever after, he enjoys his walks to and from school. He never gets to the point of liking the well, but any feelings of anxiety are fleeting because *he's looked down the abyss and survived.*

If fear is keeping you from obtaining knowledge about some aspect of your illness, try putting your full attention on the problem that frightens you most and talking your way through to answers that work. For me, my greatest fear was that my children's lives would be ruined by having to grow up without me. This fear could have become like the deep well, distracting me with its terribleness. Fortunately, a colleague, Steve, visited me in the hospital the day after my diagnosis. After a perfunctory "How are you?" Steve cut to the chase: "Wendy, what do you fear most?" I stammered, "Dying, and my kids not having a mom." Instead of offering the usual platitudes and steering me away from such thoughts, Steve stabbed the heart of my fear, prodding me with direct questions such as "What would happen to them? Would they be abandoned on a street corner? Go to school? Would they grow up and be happy?" In making me realize that, as awful as it would be, they would survive and thrive in the loving care of remaining family and friends, he helped me put boundaries around my greatest fear. Each time my cancer recurred and my fears for my children resurfaced, I automatically tapped into my belief that they would be fine—different, but still healthy and happy. This comforting and inspiring belief was born when I looked at what I feared most and found an answer that alleviated this fear.

Your personal deep, dark well may be fear of pain, debility, abandonment, poverty, death, or something else. You may not even be sure what it is you fear, but you know that it is keeping you from obtaining information about survivorship that might help. Hold the hand of someone who can support you as you look at what you fear most. Loosen fear's grip on you. In the company of knowledgeable and caring people, face your fears that are keeping you from information and inspiration that might help.

What are the things you fear most? Is there someone who can help you deal with them?

Taming Symptom-Related Fears

Physical symptoms often trigger fear that can range from crisp images of specific illness-related horrors to free-floating generalized anxiety that you may not even connect in your mind with the symptom causing it. Fears roaming through your head such as "It might be this" and "What if it's that?" can drain your strength even though any one fear at any one moment may seem insignificant. In most cases, talking with your health-care team about your worrisome symptom puts boundaries around your fears of what might be wrong.

In chapter 5, I told the story of a middle-aged man who develops a dry cough after completing radiation therapy for lung cancer. He tries to ignore the cough, and he delays seeing his doctor for fear the cough is caused by his cancer returning. Although avoiding evaluation allows him to avoid bad news in the short run, his racking cough forces him to keep wrestling with a host of fears such as "I might have cancer again. I might need treatment again. I might be sick from treatment and lose my job, and, and, and . . ." With his imagination unchecked, fears kept feeding more fears. When he ultimately visits his doctor, he learns that his cancer is still in remission and he has a common, treatable aftereffect of radiation.

A mind game that calms my fears when I have a worrisome test result or symptom is this: *Do the right thing while planning on a good outcome.* While visiting my doctor and while undergoing evaluation, I focus on all the minor problems it might be. Unlike patients who use this tactic to reassure themselves ("It's probably nothing serious") while avoiding evaluation, I can wholeheartedly focus on good outcomes because I am taking the right steps not to miss the serious possibilities. Fostering my positive emotions —in this case, my hope that I'll be fine and my confidence that knowledge (even bad news) is power—helps me get good care and feel better.

Is your fear helping you or hurting you?

Calming Fear from Upsetting News

What if the news is bad? What if the man in chapter 5 found out he did have cancer again? Yes, he'd likely be upset, but he could also experience elements of relief ("I don't have to wonder and worry anymore") and motivation ("Let's figure out what to do to help this situation"). If the goal is to minimize problems and be as healthy as possible, he could calm his fear by focusing on the value of the upsetting-but-useful information, recognizing that a period of increased stress is often associated with getting something you want. Think back to times in your life when you expected and accepted distress to reach a goal. For me, going through medical school and delivering my babies are experiences that immediately come to my mind. When something is precious, it is worth the pain and sacrifice needed to obtain it. Learning the truth about your condition is an important goal because the truth can help you, even if it makes you unhappy now.

> The truth can help you, even if it makes you unhappy when you discover it.

Reframing—seeing your problem in a different light—may help tame your fears. After enduring months of treatment-related discomforts and distress to get my cancer into remission, my suffering from fear of recurrence felt like salt on a wound. So I reframed my anxiety as "a luxury reserved for people in remission," and I no longer resented the fear. Almost magically, I felt less fearful, too.

Tips to Tame Fears

- Focus your attention on factors under your control (e.g., healthful diet, proper exercise, taking therapies properly, working well with your health-care team, obtaining support).
- Distract yourself from the source of your fear.

- Reframe your fear.
- Practice self-relaxation or self-hypnosis.
- Talk to yourself in positive, hopeful ways.
- Get counseling.
- Pray.

You can learn a wide variety of techniques for taming fear from counselors, clergy, support groups, self-help books and Web sites, and your health-care team. Different approaches may work for you in different situations, or for similar situations at different times. The more techniques you know, the more tools you have available to help you tame fears and live well with the fear that remains.

*How often does a desire to avoid something upsetting keep
you from obtaining knowledge about your situation?
What techniques are you using to calm your fears?
Who is helping you calm your fears?*

Worry

Worry is a feeling of uneasiness or concern about something distressing. In contrast to fear, which you feel in reaction to imminent threat, worry can be in response to problems that are not frightening or imminent. As with any emotion, worry that prompts you to take positive action is good, as long as you stop worrying once you've responded. One of the lesser-used definitions of worry is "to seize something with the teeth and shake or tug repeatedly," as, for example, a dog worrying a bone. If you find yourself worrying, ask yourself, "Is my worrying helping me in any way, or am I just wearing myself out like a dog shaking a bone?"

If worry is becoming your new way of life, remember:

1. Problems that never materialized didn't happen! So, stop worrying about them. Why worry about a potential complication of past treat-

ment that never occurred? You wouldn't worry about it raining on your outdoor picnic if the gathering was yesterday and you ate under sunny skies.

2. Potential problems are nothing more than possibilities for the future that may never come to be. Find out what you can do to decrease the likelihood of problems, and then stop worrying. Once you are doing what you can to prevent problems, there is no good in worrying about it.

3. Today's problems are beyond worry. You wouldn't worry about failing an exam if you were holding your test paper with an "F" on it. The bad news is that you already have the problem you worried about. The good news is you can stop worrying and shift your focus to solutions and adjustments that will help you move beyond the problem.

Which of your worries are about concerns beyond your control?
How can you use your worrying to help you get good care?

Pink Elephants

Worries keep you from fully enjoying today. If you let go of worry, the associated unpleasant emotions usually fade, too. The problem is that you may find it hard to shake off illness-related worries because your worries are not shared by most people, and because many worries may be new to you. Harness your mind's tremendous ability to protect you. Learn ways for dealing with thoughts that are harmful to your well-being. Simple repression (mental blocking out) of your knowledge of unpleasant facts may work best for you. This technique is not unique to extraordinary people who are adept at mind control. All day long you forget about the risks you take. Otherwise you'd be crazy with worry every time you got in a car or ate in a restaurant. So, you see, you already know how to block out knowledge of potential problems. Have confidence in your ability to let go of worry related to your illness. Try telling yourself "I'm not going to think about it." You may need to develop some phrases that help you to disengage from the worry. Some of my personal favorites include

- "I *refuse* to let worry steal an otherwise good time!"
- "Thinking about that isn't helping me";
- "Tomorrow I'll worry about tomorrow";
- "Why worry?" (I am usually picturing the philosophizing *Mad* magazine character Alfred E. Newman while I say this.)

Unfortunately, emotionally charged thoughts are not like light switches that you can turn on and off at will. Telling you to put something upsetting out of your mind may feel like I'm asking you to forget a terrible secret you wish you hadn't been told. Or, it may seem like the prank "For the next three minutes you are allowed to think about anything you want *except pink elephants*." Of course, for the next few minutes or hours, all you can think about are pink elephants.

If you can't shut off the thoughts, find a distraction to focus on. Turn to activities that always engage your attention, calm you, or bring you joy such as gardening, reading a book, watching a good movie, exercising, making or listening to music, dancing, or working on your computer. Worry beads, touching stones, prayer, exercise, rest, and meditation are tools that may help calm your anxiety and allow you to shift your attention to life-enhancing thoughts and activities.

A different approach is to *use* your worry, transforming worthless worry into heightened appreciation for the good things today. This is a twist on the old adage that you don't know what you have until it's gone. For example, my premature osteoporosis puts me at risk for bone fracture. Having cared for many patients with fractures, I have a good idea of the trauma this can entail. Instead of dwelling on the troubles a fracture would bring, I revel in my current mobility and freedom from hip and back pain. Gratitude for what you have comes naturally to some people; for others, it is a learned behavior that comes only after time and practice.

Yet another trick to taming anxiety about the future is to emphasize the uncertainty. "I know the statistical risks for someone in my situation, but nobody knows for sure exactly what the future holds *for me.*" Don't despair if you are still worrying despite attempts at repression, distraction, and reframing. Discuss this with your doctors and nurses. They need to know you are worrying. Exaggerated anxiety can be related to your medical condition, your medications, an underlying anxiety disorder, or other treatable problems. In the meantime, keep trying the techniques. You may just need more time.

What methods help you tame your anxiety when you find out about potential problems? Have you discussed your worries and worrying with your health-care team?

Grief

I was in my chemo-nurse's office, crying, when I mentioned how I appreciated my oncologist's expert care. Brenda responded, "He wishes you weren't so sad." It touched me deeply to know he didn't want me hurting emotionally, but her comment also took me by surprise. I knew I was afraid (dealing with recurrent cancer and a worsening prognosis) and stressed (trying to make difficult decisions about treatments), but I didn't realize how sad I was. Once she said it, the floodgates opened.

I had more than enough reasons to feel sad. I'd just spent hours at my office, selling my medical equipment and referring my patients to other physicians. The emotional trauma of closing my medical practice was the backdrop to my illness-associated losses: loss of physical comfort as I underwent biopsies and scans; loss of ability to work; loss of confidence in my future. My normal routines were going to be disrupted for months, at best. My identity as a healthy doctor (or, at any rate, a recuperating doctor) was transformed to "doctor with cancer." Worst of all, I'd lost any sense of control of my world.

All patients sustain losses. The human reaction to loss is grief. Usually experienced as a heavy feeling in the chest and a change in appetite and sleep pattern, grief can masquerade as anger, apathy, and a host of other emotions and physical symptoms. Grief is not pure sadness, either. It can be sadness mixed with anger, jealousy, guilt, fear, and shame. Although each person's grief is unique, one thing is shared: Grief hurts. There is no pill or magic way to bypass the grief process for all our little and big losses. But grief heals.

Patients who don't realize they are grieving might mistakenly attribute their symptoms as due to their illness, thus adding to their burden of worries and fears. Patients whose sadness is downplayed or discouraged by others feel bad about their sadness, which only complicates a difficult time. A young patient was flustered by her well-intentioned but insensitive friends and family who admonished,

Healthy grief is part of the landscape of Healthy Survivorship.

"Don't feel sad about losing your breast. Your *life* is what matters!" Of course her life is far more important. And she would make the same sacrifice again. Yet hers was a real and painful loss that deserves to be respected and needs to be grieved. It was only after grieving my loss of energy that I could feel truly happy within the physical limitations that define my days. Embrace your grief, and immerse yourself in its healing powers by talking with friends, family, a support group, or a counselor about your losses. Explore different ways to grieve such as journaling, art, or music. *Use* your grief to move forward. Lean on people who can comfort and support you through your grief work.

You are not the only one grieving. Although the disease or injury happened to you, your illness experience affects all those people involved in your life, especially those who love you. It helps when they recognize that they are experiencing their own crises and losses, and therefore grief.

From a more philosophical point of view, loss is part of the human condition and is often a necessary part of healthy growth. Pruning tree branches in the fall encourages luxurious flowering in the spring. Painful childbirth brings forth our precious children. Your unwanted losses may open a path to heightened joy and meaning in your life, as will be explored in chapter 10. Take comfort in knowing that getting through painful grief can help you heal and recapture joy in your life. Use your grief to help you grow.

What losses have you sustained? How do you express your grief? Who can support you through your grief?

Downtime

When dealing with serious illness, you most likely will have moments or hours or days when you are upset, irritable, and unfocused. Nothing you or anyone else can say or do will make you feel happy. I remember well the morning when my husband and I met with my oncologist to discuss treatment options for my second recurrence. I was sitting in his office, taking deep breaths and pinching the bridge of my nose in a vain attempt to keep my tears from falling. My doctor stopped talking and tenderly handed me a box of tissues. The three of us listened to me sniffle and blow my nose. When I realized that my doctor was going to wait until my distress abated before resuming our discussion of my treatment options, I looked up at him and croaked through that crazy mixture of giggles and grief, "You can keep talking. I'm not a blithering idiot. I'm just blithering!"

My usual style of curbing fear, sadness, or anxiety was to charge headlong into obtaining knowledge about the next step in my evaluation or treatment. Other times, I responded with a flare-up of the nesting instinct, cleaning out my closets or busily occupying myself with other productive but non-cancer-related chores at home. But on occasion the stress of illness got to me, and I couldn't read, write, or do much of anything. What helped more than anything else was just to acknowledge "Today is a bad day" and give myself permission to wallow in downtime. Aptly expressed by a woman who'd valiantly tolerated years of treatment, "I have days when I just can't put on my game face." On down days, instead of trying to feel or act brave, I proudly wear my colorful lapel pin that says "Cancer Sucks!" I might call someone who won't feel obligated to cheer me up, and we'll talk freely about all the ways I am feeling unhappy. If everyone is busy, I'll settle down on the sofa and pop a sappy movie in the VCR. Alternatively, I'll escape all the seriousness by indulging in "retail therapy." Off to the mall I go (preferably without my credit card). On the really bad days, I've been known to say, "Forget it, I'm going to bed!" Sleeping is a healthy way to take control, knowing I'll start a fresh day tomorrow with renewed energy and hope. When things are rough, you may need to give yourself permission to feel low for a while.

I have two warnings. First, don't slip into feeling sorry for yourself. Some survivors think it helps to indulge in pity parties every once in a while, but I see them as a dangerous invitation to a downward spiral of hopelessness and despair. Feeling sad and worn out is one thing; feeling self-pity is another. (Of course, if you find that pity parties help you, then go ahead.) Second, whether you have downtime for a few hours or a whole day or two, keep it limited. Don't let it keep you too long from obtaining useful information and doing what you need to do. If you feel stuck, get help. The goal is to get to the point where you can focus on potential solutions and finding happiness.

How do you relieve sadness? What are the best things for you to do when you are down? How often do you let yourself have a bad day and not try to be "up"?

Anger

Anger is a strong feeling of displeasure that can manifest itself as overt hostility or as passive-aggressiveness, helplessness, and other feelings. A normal response to a perceived threat, injustice, or irritation, your anger is often mixed with other emotions. It may also be the outward expression of your grief. You may have justified anger about the reaction of certain people to your illness or about some aspect of your medical care. The object of your ire may be more abstract, such as outrage at the unfairness of life.

The key question is this: What are you going to do with your anger? Bottled up anger drains energy and can interfere with your important relationships, especially when it slips out as irritability, sadness, sarcasm, or hypercritical remarks. One sick dad was so nasty to his wife and young children that he made a bad situation worse for himself and the people he loved most, leaving a legacy of wounds. Expressing anger is a disaster if the way you do so hurts others or yourself.

If you are feeling anger, ask yourself "Is my anger helping me or hurting me?" Instead of *directing* your anger at the people who care for and about you, *share* your anger with those who can listen and help. Obviously, if you're bothered by a problem that is fixable, the best way to resolve your anger is to repair the problem. You may need the assistance of friends, family, and your health-care team to resolve the problem. If these people can't help, or your problem is not reparable, try talking through your feelings with friends, journaling, or nonverbal expression like art, music, exercise, or sports.

You may need to talk with a counselor. Jeanne is a car-accident survivor whose family constantly urged her to stifle her anger. Jeanne sought relief in the office of a social worker. Professionals are more objective, trained to help you understand the source of your fury and to teach you anger-management techniques. If you've been wronged in some way, forgiveness plays a central role in your healing. Forgiving someone in your heart frees you from the anger that is hurting you more than anyone else.

You might do best not quieting your anger but, instead, mobilizing it toward useful actions. One shy patient I know, distraught over his diagnosis and the hopeless prognosis given to him by the first doctor who evaluates him, seeks a second opinion. The new specialist tells him of promising clinical trials for people with his illness, igniting the patient's rage at the first doctor, who had closed the book on hope without ever consulting other experts. Now the patient is a man on a mission. With his fist in the air and an "I'll show you!" attitude, his anger fuels the fortitude and hopefulness he needs to travel for consultations and treatments. He assembles a group of supporters, eats without an appetite, and does his exercises when he feels tired. This man feels fully alive, the power of his anger channeled into useful activity. Use the power of anger in healthy ways.

What or who is making you angry? What can you do to dispel your anger? How can you channel the energy of your anger in ways that help you?

Guilt

You should feel guilty only if you did something wrong. It is not uncommon to feel guilty for doing well when someone else with a similar disease is doing poorly, or to feel uncomfortable for surviving while others succumb—so-called survivor's guilt. But since your recovery did not cause their troubles, you have no reason to feel guilty. It also doesn't make sense to feel guilty about your genetic makeup if you have a hereditary condition or about landing on the bad side of the statistics if you develop a complication of treatment. If you didn't do anything wrong, let guilt go.

What if you feel guilty because you are partly responsible for your current situation, like the patient who smoked cigarettes or ignored early warning signs before developing a heart attack or cancer? If past choices *may* have contributed to your current medical problems, recognize the uncertainty. People without your risk factors get sick, too; it is possible you would have developed your problem anyway. Forgive yourself for past mistakes that may have contributed to your illness. Remember: You are human. Transform your guilt into motivation to repair a problem, such as to stop smoking or to report symptoms early from now on.

What if you've forgiven yourself and made positive changes but still can't let go of guilt? For you, feelings of guilt may arise every time you see your loved ones dealing with the consequences of your past poor choices. Guilt is not helping anyone, here. You may be able to let go of guilt if you ask yourself "Was I trying to get sick?" For example, did you smoke cigarettes *with the intention of getting sick and hurting your family*? The answer most certainly is "no." Forgive yourself your imperfections and move on.

What if other people are making you feel guilty? Accusations such as "If you hadn't smoked so much, you wouldn't feel crummy now!" can make it hard for you not to feel responsible for all the problems. More subtle hints of disapproval can eat away at your confidence and trust, too. These tensions need to be addressed. They rarely go away by themselves, and they poison the atmosphere for healing and finding joy. Acknowledge others' feelings, and then explain the effect on you of their comments. Remind them that you never tried to get sick, and that you are trying to get better now. Ask them how you can move forward, together. If needed, have a third party help them understand and forgive you, so they can let go of bad feelings and embrace you with love.

The stickiest and most debilitating situations can occur when your ongoing choices are hurting your health. Maybe you skip doses of your medications to save money, or maybe you repeatedly delay medical appointments to avoid missing work. If you smoke cigarettes, drink alcohol, take recreational drugs, or eat an unhealthy diet, your family may struggle to respond to your illness in supportive ways. In extreme cases, a patient's unhealthy behavior becomes a central issue that tears the family apart. On the one hand, your loved ones want to be loving and sympathetic. After all, you are sick and vulnerable. On the other hand, they may feel so angry and disappointed, frustrated, or hurt that they can't deal with you in helpful ways. From their point of view, how can they wholeheartedly join your team for recovery when they feel that you are still hurting your health?

If you feel guilty or if your loved ones remain angry at you, go together for counseling. An impartial professional can help you work through the anger and guilt that are taking the focus away from physical and emotional healing.

What do you feel guilty about? If you did something that may have contributed to your illness, how can you go about forgiving yourself?

Disappointment, Jealousy, Annoyance, Regret, and Other Negative Emotions

You can be dragged down or lifted up by disappointment, jealousy, annoyance, regret, and other unpleasant emotions. Imagine that you are having one setback after another, and another patient is responding extremely well to the same treatment you are receiving or is having an easy time with treatment that is knocking you flat. Jealousy could cause you to cancel your follow-up appointment and feel hopeless. Jealousy could also prompt you to request an earlier follow-up appointment, hopeful of making adjustments that help. If, in another scenario, you made a judgment error regarding the significance of some recent symptoms, your sense of regret can diminish your self-confidence if you beat up on yourself, or boost your self-confidence by motivating you to learn from past mistakes. More important than what you feel is what you do with what you are feeling.

Which emotions are making you feel bad about yourself? About others? About your future or the world? Are you feeling unlucky? Singled out? Alone? Misunderstood? Are your emotions making you unhappy or happy? You decide what you do with your unpleasant emotions. Don't let them make you bitter. Use them in hopeful and purposeful ways that bring you healing and joy.

What other unpleasant emotions are you experiencing? Are they helping you or hurting you? Who can help you use them in healthy ways?

Emotions and Limits

In chapter 4, I discussed the challenges associated with your fluctuating limits as you go through treatment and recovery. Even when your limits are pretty obvious, your emotions can complicate simple matters. For instance, my surgeon stated clearly in his discharge instructions that I should not lift anything heavier than twenty pounds until he removed my stitches. The evening after I got home from the hospital, I took a walk around the block with Will, my then twenty-three-pound toddler. He tripped and started crying. For a host of emotional reasons—maternal instinct, desire to feel in control, disbelief and denial about my diagnosis, sadness at all I was losing, anger at my new limits—I picked him up. My husband went ballistic, which upset me, which upset him and the rest of the family.

Throughout my survivorship, anytime I tried to extend myself beyond my ability, my whole family suffered the ripple effect of my poor performance and my fatigue and irritability afterward. Then I'd feel frustrated, ashamed and guilty, angry, or just plain stupid. Medical knowledge helped me know my limits; knowledge about my emotions helped me respect them.

Are you experiencing any feelings of anger, disappointment, jealousy, annoyance, regret, or guilt? For each feeling, is it helping you get good care? Is it helping you live more fully? How can you use the feeling to your advantage? If the feeling is only hurting you, what can you do to let it go?

Healthy Denial

Confusion arises when people talk about denial. This term is used loosely in our society, meaning anything from maladaptive denial to healthy repression of painful truths. Technically speaking, *denial* is an abnormal refusal to accept the truth. If Roger can't walk due to a broken bone, and he says, "My leg is perfectly fine," he is in denial. In contrast to denial, *repression* is the unconscious exclusion of painful impulses, desires, or fears

> Denial can help you enjoy today in the face of tomorrow's uncertainty.

from your conscious mind. If, while driving to the hospital, Roger calmly reassures his family, "It's probably nothing," he is repressing, not denying, the possibility that his leg is broken. Ask him what bad news they could find, and he will tell you, "An X ray will show if it's broken."

Usually, when people suggest you are "in denial," they say it in a derogatory tone, as if you are better off perceiving your world in a thoroughly factually accurate way at all times. Let me assure you that without denial I couldn't get good care or be happy. Although one of my fundamental beliefs is that the truth will set me free, well-used repression is indispensable to my Healthy Survivorship. Denial helped me pursue risky treatments in 1993 and 1994 that got me better.

While rotating through the cancer ward as a medical student, I was concerned about an elderly patient who, because of her cultural upbringing, was ashamed of her breast cancer. She talked about her medicines (chemotherapy) as good treatment for her "little infection." Whenever someone in the oncology clinic asked what type of cancer she had, she said that her doctor, an oncologist, treated many patients like her who never had cancer. I was baffled by the staff's willingness to play along with her denial until I realized that her denial was the only way this patient would get good care. Unable to let go of lifelong beliefs, similar patients in her community avoided embarrassment by declining effective treatment.

Denial is fine as long as it is not keeping you from a truth that can help you. Denying worrisome symptoms keeps you from needed medical care that can help. Denying that you are struggling emotionally (or socially, spiritually, or financially) when, in fact, things are rocky, keeps you from opportunities for improved well-being and growth. How do you know if your denial may be a problem? One major clue is that you find yourself disagreeing with your doctors and close family members about the most basic aspects of your care, such as your need for treatment or how much you are eating. Talk with an objective third party such as a social worker, nurse, or other member of your health-care team. A professional can be your advocate, validating your healthy use of denial or guiding you to a more balanced approach if your denial is hurting you.

> Denial is fine as long as it is not keeping you from a truth that can help you. Denial is fine as long as you are doing what you need to do to get good care.

The flip side of maladaptive denial—namely, an unhealthy focus on harsh facts—is a potential obstacle to Healthy Survivorship as well. If your imagination conjures "disaster" with every tiny ache or pain, ring of your phone, or routine checkup, you've lost your ability for healthy denial. At least, for now. Give yourself time to adjust to your illness. Your healthy wall of denial can rebuild itself, especially if you recover completely, although it may never be quite as solid as it was before your diagnosis. If your ability to push worrisome thoughts or fears out of your mind does not improve over time, ask your health-care team for referral to someone who can teach you relaxation techniques and healthy ways of thinking about what worries you. Support-group members, counselors, and clergy may be able to help you regain a healthy sense of denial to live well in uncertain times.

How are you using denial at this time? Is denial helping you or hurting you?

When Life Feels Unreal

Life can feel unreal when you have discord between what you understand rationally and what feels normal or familiar to you as you go about your day. Anytime you are experiencing something new, it can feel unreal—especially if unexpected, but even when you have been planning for it. It doesn't matter if it is your first few days of high school or after losing a loved one. Usually, as the situation becomes more familiar through experience, you develop a "new normal" that includes the changes; it feels real, no matter what is actually happening. Talking, writing letters, journaling, and reading about your situation may help you get to the new normal that includes your illness.

A little bit of unreality is common, and not a problem by itself. More than a month after my diagnosis, I wrote a letter to a cousin that she shared with me a few years later. I'd written all about starting chemotherapy and closing my office. My letter went on to describe the new routine of my days—chemo, taking care of my kids, trying to eat, trying to sleep—and my insights, hopes, and strategies for handling all the challenges. Clearly I was dealing fairly well with the tangible changes in my life and adjusting to my diagnosis. Reading on, my postscript took me by surprise: "P.S. I still have this feeling that I'll wake up and find this is all a horrible dream."

The little sense of unreality can last indefinitely. One woman in a support group had been dealing with recurrent ovarian cancer for years. Besides the obvious stigmata of illness—baldness, weight loss, and bruises from intravenous lines—she was dealing with pain and fatigue on a daily basis. With her scans showing relentless progression of her disease, she understood the gravity of her situation. Yet when a friend shared a letter inquiring about "your friend who is really sick with cancer," the patient was taken aback. She told us, "I can't believe that I'm someone who people think of as 'really sick with cancer.'" This disconnect between what she knew to be true and what felt real to her was not a problem. It didn't keep her from learning about her illness or doing what she needed to do to try to get better. Her repression and sense of unreality were adaptive, keeping her grief and fear at bay so that she could enjoy what she had.

My Emotions—Your Emotions

A sense of unreality may make the stress easier to handle at times, especially at first, but you will find the stress of serious illness very real. And stress affects emotions. Throughout my survivorship, I've had times when I've been more emotional than usual. My family members have been more emotional, too. Illness is a challenge that can rouse everyone's emotions in different ways at different times. It helps to remember an obvious truism: Only I can feel what I feel. And I can't feel what others are feeling. This is a gap that can't be eliminated, only bridged. Healthy Survivorship means doing what I can to meet partway the people who care and want to help.

When you are sick, you don't need others' sympathy. You don't need them to *feel* what you are feeling. What you need is for the important people in your life to know what's going on with you. It's up to you to help that happen. If I want my husband to know that I'm particularly exhausted that evening, I do best to say, "Hon, I'm too tired to make dinner tonight," even though I think it should be obvious from my two long naps in the afternoon. So, too, if Ted expects me to be sensitive to his need for quiet time to prepare a lec-

> Only you can feel what you feel, and that's okay.

ture, he may have to tell me, "I need to be left alone in my study for a few hours," even though I've seen him prepare lectures for years.

Your emotional needs should be clear, too. Those who care for you need to know if you are feeling anxious about an upcoming checkup or sad about missing a social event. It's a bonus if they *understand* why you're feeling the way you do. My best friend once said, "Wendy, I really don't understand why you feel the way you do, but I believe you do and will help you any way I can." Help yourself by helping others know what mood you are in. You might have to experiment to find the best way to talk about emotions. Ted and I finally devised a pact: Steel ourselves and tell it like it is. "Ted, I'm angry about . . . and I need to talk (or, I need to cool down by going for a walk)." This way, Ted doesn't wonder why I'm acting the way I am or assume he's doing something to make me mad.

The stress of family illness may make you and those around you less sensitive to others' needs. You may have trouble communicating needs for the first time in your relationship. Counselors can help you communicate well while under stress and prevent molehill problems from growing into mountainous ones. Under the best of circumstances, breakdowns in communication are unavoidable and people get hurt. Forgiveness brings healing, enabling everyone to refocus on efforts that bring joy.

Emotions are contagious, in a way. You may need to separate yourself somewhat from people who are going through a rough spell or aren't coping well. Being around someone who is depressed can be downright depressing. Seeing fear in your partner's eyes can trigger or heighten your own anxiety. If my husband is having a bad day, I'm not helping him, me, or my kids if I lose my zest or feel guilty about feeling cheerful. I love Ted and care that he's unhappy, but I need to respond in helpful ways without getting sucked into a bad mood myself. Encourage others not to let your down moods affect them adversely, either. Tell them they can care and be supportive, without feeling sympathy or feeling that they are responsible for fixing your mood.

What about all the bad stuff going on in the world around you? How do you keep from feeling despair about the wars, fires, child abductions, accidents, and natural disasters reported on the news? Should you shield yourself? It depends. If discussing other troubles makes it harder for you to deal with your illness, you should learn as much or as little as you want, and not dwell on any of it. At times, you may do best to avoid it. When Steven Spielberg's movie about the holocaust, *Schindler's List*, was released during one of my recurrences, steering clear of the vivid dramatization of injustice and suffering seemed the better part of valor. My family went to the theater without me.

Should other people protect you from their troubles? A hard-and-fast rule doesn't work. When your emotional reserves are stretched by illness, you'll have times when you need to minimize involvement with outside troubles. Learning about others' tribulations may be the last straw, making you feel overwhelmed or despairing. Other times, learning about and dealing with others' troubles may be good for you. As will be discussed in chapter 10, caring about another can lift you up and away from your own troubles. Hearing about others' troubles may give you new perspective about your illness, making you feel less alone, less afraid, and less angry or sad.

If a crisis hits close to home, choosing to avoid the additional emotional stress means isolating yourself from your loved ones. Why work so hard to survive, only to avoid living? Get additional support so you can continue to heal while going through a terribly tough set of circumstances. These are times when you can't be upbeat or happy; you just have to find a way through the crisis.

How are you helping others know what you are feeling and what you need? How well are you in tune with others' feelings and needs? How much do you want to deal with others' problems today?

Shifting Roles/Shifting Perspectives

You learn through experience what helps you heal in your different relationships. For me, on those days when I'm not feeling particularly well physically, I still enjoy socializing with friends—if I don't talk about my medical situation when I don't want to. If someone asks me how I'm doing, I answer "fine" no matter what is going on. I've found that downplaying or diverting attention away from my discomforts helps me feel happier. I've realized that, as long as I am keeping the important people in my life aware of what is happening medically, I don't have to always give detailed (or honest) answers about my condition if doing so drags me down.

This coping style that is advantageous to me in social situations would hurt me in medical situations. I am with my doctors for only a relatively short period of time; they need me to be forthright so they can know exactly what is going on with me. Doctor appointments are not social visits. For my doctors to be able to help me, I have to shift into patient mode and answer the question "How are you?" as accurately as possible. I used to leave my oncologist's office feeling a little bit blue, even when things were going relatively well. That's because I'd rather say "I'm fine" just as I do in social situations, instead of talking about my weaknesses and ongoing difficulties. Ever since I understood what was going on with my emotions, my confidence that I am helping my recovery with honest answers has overshadowed the blue feeling. And once I leave my doctor's office, I shift right back into the style that helps me in social situations.

When you are with your loved ones, you need them to know what's going on with you, too. But you are with them often, and they don't need to know every little thing every little second. As a Healthy Survivor, determine how much to focus on your illness at any given time. When you are with your friends, you have to figure out how much you want to say, and when. My friends and I have an understanding: If they ask me "How are you?" I'll respond in whatever way works for me, trusting that the person wants to "be there," whatever "be there" means at that minute. With my answer, I share the truth about survival: Some days are good, some bad;

sometimes I need to escape, sometimes I need to talk it all out, sometimes I need to be held, other times I need space, and I'm not always sure what I need, so they can't know, either. Honesty and effort lead to healing relationships.

Tips on Illness and Relationships

- *My illness*, not me, is causing others' distress; I am not responsible for their distress.
- Relationships change in changing situations, and that's okay.
- More than anything else, people who care about me want me to do *what I need to do* to get better and feel better, even if it is not what they would want.
- Sometimes it is hard for anyone to know what I am supposed to be doing (and not doing) at the moment.
- If I tell others what I need and don't need, they can do a better job of helping me.
- Relationships can't be perfect; they can be real.
- Forgiveness is healing.

What do you need from each of your relationships? What can you do to make these relationships work well? Who can help you if you are having trouble with a relationship?

Emotions and Support

For me, seeking, using, and sharing medical information was a knee-jerk response to my predicament that provided me a sense of escape from the prison of my illness. Seeking and accepting practical and emotional support, however, charted unfamiliar and terribly uncomfortable territory. At first, I saw asking for help with anything from my home responsibilities to my uncomfortable emotions as evidence of yet more areas of loss of control, and a sure sign of weakness. As a Healthy Survivor, seeking and accepting help demonstrates strength and allows you to regain some control. Accepting assistance frees your energy and attention for healing. Life is too short to refuse help when help can make your life better and happier.

Picture this in your mind: You are trying to climb a mountain wearing a backpack filled with both necessities and rocks. To get to the top as safely and comfortably as possible, what do you do? You empty the rocks and carry a lighter load. Lighten the load of your illness—the practical and emotional stresses—by getting needed guidance and support when struggling with pain or other medical problems, intense emotions, and home or work responsibilities. Demands on your time, energy, and emotions are much more manageable when shared.

If you don't like being a "taker," keep in mind that when you accept others' assistance, whether it is help with the practical demands of your illness or the emotional strain on you, you are *giving* others opportunities to feel fulfilled. And, if you get help, you lift the spirits of those who care about you by allowing them to do something that helps you feel better or get better. I suppose I could have survived my treatments without accepting any help from friends and neighbors and without all those counseling sessions with the oncology social worker. But it would have been harder on everyone I cared about. I'm sure that I got through the hard times more smoothly because of help. I also learned about myself, including some things I didn't particularly like or feel proud of, but that were useful in knowing how to handle situations. Counseling and support helped me grow as a person through my illness. I

> When you are sick, accepting help is one way to gain control.

believe I was happier than I would have been without the help, and I'm definitely happier now because of it. If your reluctance to accept help reflects a desire to remain in control, think about this: When you are sick, letting go and accepting help is one way to gain control. Be conscious of not allowing a desire for control keep you from assistance that can help your recovery.

Leaning on others and sharing your enlightened and noble thoughts, as well as the frightening and embarrassing ones, will help everyone

understand and deal with what is happening. Sharing helps you release
tensions and see whatever is happening in life-enhancing ways. Sharing
helps you deal with your reality even when you can't change what's happening. Just because you *can* get through without help doesn't mean you
should.

*What kind of support would help you? Who can provide
support?*

Emotions and Money

Some experts on relationships claim that most people would rather talk
about sexual problems or death than money! Money matters, especially
when you have medical needs. Even under relatively good conditions—
you have medical insurance, and you aren't going to lose your job or
home—finances can become an emotional third rail. I'm thinking of one
particular couple whose emotions are keeping them from talking about
the financial burden of his expensive medical treatments. The tedious
and time-consuming job of paying the pile of medical bills is confusing
to the husband, and upsetting in ways that paying heating bills aren't. He
feels vulnerable and out of control ("I don't know what half the things
listed on my bill are, so how can I know if my bill is correct?") as well as
embarrassed. While he feels guilty that savings intended for a vacation
are now being used to pay his medical bills, his wife feels ashamed that
she resents the expense. When a bill for a scan done on a particular date-
of-service arrives in the mail, she also feels upset as she remembers that
awful day.

Beyond the practical budgetary problems, their decision making
about their family's savings and investments is no longer an issue of dollars and cents. How they spend (or don't spend) their money has become
a concrete expression of their sense of hopefulness (or hopelessness)
about the future, and a reminder of their many losses. Money issues have
become so emotional that they both avoid thinking or talking about

finances as much as possible, and consequently they deprive themselves of useful information that might help them financially and emotionally. As discussed in chapter 3 (pages 82–84), individuals and organizations are available to help you work through financial tensions that may be keeping you from getting good care and living fully.

What is your financial situation? Who can help you deal with stresses related to money?

Uplifting Emotions

With a watering can swinging in one hand, a mom walks over to an old-fashioned outdoor pump and says to her pigtailed daughter, "Let's fill this to the top!" They start pumping and the water level in the can rises slowly, to the young girl's delight. When almost halfway filled, the can begins sprouting leaks. Despite valiant efforts to cover all the pinholes with their fingers, the water level steadily drops. With an impish grin, the girl lets go of the can, reaches over to the handle of the water pump, and starts pumping furiously. Water rushes out of the spout, quickly filling the can to overflowing.

Negative emotions can be like the pinholes in the watering can, draining your emotional reserves despite your best efforts to either use them in positive ways or let them go. Even under the best of circumstances, dealing with illness drains physical and emotional energy needed for living. When I think back to the rough times of my survivorship, the inescapable emotions that come to mind are the ones that made me most miserable: the fear, sadness, anxiety, disappointment, guilt, and lack of confidence. But, in fact, many uplifting emotions were stirred up, too. My competitive and determined nature went into high gear. Curiosity about my upcoming medical adventure helped me the same way it had when I was six years old and needed courage to look behind the little door that my older siblings had convinced me led to the monster's house under the steps to the basement.

Don't miss opportunities for health and happiness. Learn how to fill up your emotional reservoir by turning on positive feelings. Use your positive emotions to mollify negative ones and work toward solutions. Interestingly, your negative emotions (such as anger or frustration) usually resolve once the inciting problem is resolved, while your positive emotions can linger, enhancing your life long after the challenge that prompted them has been overcome. Positive emotions can help you through and beyond hard times.

When dealing with illness, positive emotions come naturally to some people but only with great effort to others. Make an effort to build up your confidence in the ability of your treatments to control your illness and your health-care team to care for you. Take pride in your ability to deal with your stress and loss, and foster your sense of purpose by outlining your goals while going through treatment and recovery. Keep yourself motivated by staying involved with activities that interest you and bring you pleasure. Underlying everything must be a sense of hope, the topic of the next chapter.

Make a list of positive emotions that might help you. What can you do to "turn up the flow" of each of these positive emotions?

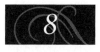

Nourishing Your Hope

I *had hope. Through the ups and downs of six months of rigorous* *chemotherapy, I remained hopeful that I would get through the treat-* *ments intact and be able to resume the usual juggling of my medical* *practice and family life. When treatment ended and my scans were clear, I* *was hopeful that the cancer was cured. Throughout my recovery, I nourished* *hopes that the lingering effects of my illness—the leg pain, sinus infections,* *and anxiety—would resolve eventually. When, eight months after returning* *to work, a new lymph node popped up in my neck, I held on to the hope that* *it was nothing more serious than a benign reaction to a recent sore throat.*

After the biopsy, my husband and I were ushered into the surgeon's con- *ference room to await the verdict. The specimen of lymph node tissue had* *been rushed to the lab for immediate diagnosis. I knew that if it showed can-* *cer, I wasn't cured. I knew that if the cancer was back, I would close my solo* *practice of medicine because months earlier, while planning on a long remis-* *sion, my husband and I had made a hard-nosed business calculation that if* *I needed to take time off work again to receive more treatment, I couldn't* *afford to keep my office open anymore.*

The call came from the pathologist, a friend of mine. After hearing the news *firsthand, I looked at my husband and made a fist with my thumb pointing straight down. As if made of oak, the door to my future slammed shut. What could I hope for now? What should I hope for? How could I find hope?*

In this chapter, I will discuss the many faces of "Healthy Hope," the roles that hope can play in healing, and the common obstacles to finding and nourishing hope. One of the most difficult challenges in becoming a Healthy Survivor is negotiating the waves of optimism and pessimism as your circumstances and outlook change over time. The goals of this chapter are to encourage you to think about your own sense of hopefulness and to find a healthy balance of hope and acceptance that works for you.

New Meaning to Hope

Hope is a natural and vital part of life. In general, hope is the belief that something you want to happen can happen. When you are very young, you might hope for a glimpse of Santa Claus on Christmas Eve, or to find a puppy (or a pony!) in your backyard the morning of your birthday. Your hopes become a bit more realistic with time, such as hoping to learn to ride your bicycle or to do well on a school exam. As you become an adult, your hopes mature, too. You may hope to meet your soulmate or to land a good job. Long-range hopes emerge that become the underpinnings of your days, such as hopes for good health, long life, success, and happiness.

When illness strikes, hope takes on new meaning. Long-held dreams may have to be postponed; some may be shattered forever. Hope that once floated quietly in the background of your consciousness now takes center stage—hope for comfort, independence, and the future. When you first learn your diagnosis, you may hope for cure and complete recovery. This desire to be healthy again is an automatic reflex. As a patient, though, it doesn't help you much by itself. Are you going to just sit there, hoping and praying that your disease disappears, instead of going to a physician? If you are in pain, out of work, or struggling to maintain important relationships strained by the demands of your illness, you may be prompted to ask what kind of hope you need.

Healthy Hope

Healthy Hope: the belief that you can help improve your
situation and feel happier

Healthy Survivors nourish a specific type of hope—Healthy Hope—
namely, the belief that you can help improve your situation and that you
can feel happier. In most cases, you help your situation by pursuing effective action, or, when the best healing salve is tincture of time, by waiting
patiently. Healthy Hope underlies your efforts to obtain knowledge about
your condition and situation, explore options, choose wisely, and then
translate possibility into reality. Even when nothing can be done to
improve what is happening, Healthy Hope shapes your perception of reality in life-enhancing ways. As taught by the ever-popular Serenity Prayer
of Reinhold Niebuhr, you can hope for the courage to change what can be
changed, the serenity to accept what cannot be changed, and the wisdom
to know the difference. Focused on the things you *can* affect or control,
you can hope for the best and, yet, be willing to take what comes.

When confronted with serious illness, Healthy Hope may not be your
initial response. Or, you may be energetically hopeful for a while after
your diagnosis, but you may lose the sense that anything you do makes a
difference after enduring the grind of evaluation and treatment or while
experiencing the reverberations of recovery or recurrence. Always
remember: In tough situations, hope does not depend on blissful ignorance or willful denial. You can cultivate genuine hope even when you are
acutely aware that things are not going well and the likelihood of a good
outcome is small. Hope is an ongoing choice.

Healing without Hope

Hope is not an absolute necessity for all patients. Depending upon your
situation, you can have times of hopelessness when you passively agree to
do whatever your physicians tell you to do. Patients have been known to
maintain a pessimistic posture while receiving treatments, and then,
when it's all over, they are cured. In many medical situations, as long as

you get effective treatment, you'll get well because the impact of treatment far overwhelms any effect of your emotional or psychological state.

So, what's the big deal about hope? For one, your quality of life during treatment is affected by your sense of hopefulness. Under the best of circumstances, it's hard to undergo unpleasant or risky treatments. Harsh treatments can be even harder when you don't have a sense that they might help you get well or feel better. For another, when your long-term recovery is iffy, factors other than choice of primary medical therapy may play a more critical role in helping your body heal than when a good outcome is assured. A nourishing diet, exercise regimen, state of mind, and good spirits may be needed to increase your odds of getting better. When the outcome feels uncertain, hope helps.

The Faces of Healthy Hope

I'm defining Healthy Hope as the belief that you can help improve your situation and feel happier. All by themselves, definitions don't always help you. For example, women who are newly pregnant for the first time are taught the definition of early labor. Yet, seven or more months later, when feeling those first contractions, they often wonder, "Is this the real thing?" In a similar way, you can know what hope is yet not recognize its presence. If you can't recognize hope, it is harder to find and nourish it. Let me try to describe the ineffable: hope.

Hope is *the mental image of your goals*. When you are facing a challenge, the hopeful picture in your mind provides a background for interpreting the objective information taken in by your senses. For example, if you are feeling miserable, you can picture your treatments repairing your problems and you can imagine feeling better than ever once you've had time to recover. Or, as you deal with strains in your relationships, you can imagine these relationships ending up stronger and richer. With hope, you can take "what is" and project "what can be." Through the lens of hope, challenges and losses are seen as opportunities to be pursued through sound knowledge and proper action. As long as your goals are realistic, these hopeful images help.

Hope is *a well of courage* during those times you feel frightened, confused, unsure, or overwhelmed. You might have times of asking "Can I do this? How do I begin?" With hope, things you thought you'd never be able to handle, somehow, now seem do-able. Hope is the feeling that you'll reach your goal, even though you may not yet know how to get where you want to go. While part of you can't believe you are doing what you're doing, you're actually doing it! As long as the course you follow is based on informed decisions, your hopeful bravery can lead toward Healthy Survivorship.

Hope is *a source of energy* that seems to defy the laws of physics. When treatments and stress wear you down, you may want to yell to the world, "No more medication. No more physicians poking or prodding me. No more bad news. I can't do it anymore!" And then, out of nowhere, comes the resolve needed to see one more physician, undergo one more test, take one more treatment, do one more exercise, or have one more discussion. "This time it may help" is the hopeful incentive of Healthy Survivors.

Peaceful waiting is another way of experiencing hope. You may feel exasperated when told, "All we can do now is wait." Ah! Waiting is so hard. But, when doing nothing is the best approach, hope makes it possible for you to let go and let your natural healing mechanisms work unhampered for a while. It is no wonder patients need patience.

You may experience hope as a feeling, sensation, thought, or sense of spirituality. You may feel it in your head, fingertips, center of your chest, or all parts of your being. When the facts about your situation pull you down and tell you "No!" hope is the spirit that lifts you up and says "Yes!" When losses make you feel like damaged goods or when pressures are breaking you, hope is the glue that makes you whole.

What do you want *to happen to you? What do you believe* can *or* will *happen to you?*

Types of Hope

Not all hope is equal. What hope you have is constructive or destructive depending on how you use it. Learn to recognize the different types of hope, and distinguish between hopes that encourage your Healthy Survivorship and those that don't.

Wishful thinking is a type of hope that is based on fantasy. Wishful hope can bring relief, comfort, and inspiration. You may enjoy daydreaming about winning the Olympics when your treatments are over. Or, you might buy a lottery ticket so you can fantasize about using the winnings for a trip around the world. This wishful thinking can help you through challenging times. The danger arises when wishful thinking keeps you from pursuing opportunities to improve your situation. Wishing for worrisome symptoms to go away on their own *instead* of reporting them to your doctors is a hope that can hurt you. Wanting your family members who have responded poorly to every earlier crisis to rise to the occasion of your illness leaves you vulnerable to disappointment and inaction. Be aware of the dangers, and use wishful thinking in healthy ways.

Blind hope is an unquestioning belief in someone or something based on unearned trust. Blind hope is appealing because it allows you to let go of responsibility and feel completely hopeful for whatever it is you want. The problem with blind hope is that it leaves no room for doubts or questions. Blind hope may lead you away from a truth that could help heal you.

Empty hope is the appearance of hopefulness for others' benefit, a façade not supported by genuine feelings. Empty hope leads toward Healthy Survivorship when it provides an outline that you can fill in with Healthy Hope as you move forward. Or, it can lead you away from Healthy Survivorship when it becomes a wall that keeps out hope that helps.

False hope is an unfounded expectation. You are hoping for something that cannot possibly come true. It can make you feel better for a while, but it comes at a price: Any attention and energy directed toward false hope is unavailable for pursuing goals that are within reach. As long as you are putting your trust in a charlatan, you are not getting effective treatments that might help. Besides the time and expense, it takes a lot of energy to maintain false hope when evidence of the truth suggests otherwise. False hope always leads you away from Healthy Survivorship and disappoints in the end.

Realistic hope is belief in the possible. Since it is based on facts, realistic hope is strong.

Faithful hope is the belief in something that is beyond your control and unable to be tested or proven. When long-standing faith is lost in the setting of illness, the void can pull you down. When spiritual faith is found or strengthened, this hope complements realistic hope by helping you address the mysteries unanswered by science. Spiritual faith does not compete with Healthy Hope as defined below. You can simultaneously let go *and* take control as expressed in the ancient Jewish saying "Pray as if everything depends on God, and act as if everything depends on you."

> Any attention or energy directed toward false hope is unavailable for pursuing goals that are within reach.

Healthy hope is the belief that your situation can improve. Realistic hope and faithful hope form the foundation of Healthy Hope. For the rest of this book, I am referring to Healthy Hope when I talk of hope, unless stated otherwise.

How much of your hope is blind hope, empty hope, false hope, realistic hope, faithful hope, and healthy hope? How can you differentiate among them?

A Hopeful Starting Stance

A hopeful starting stance is best for confronting any medical challenge. When my oncologist left my hospital room after breaking the news that I had lymphoma, my husband, Ted, and I hugged each other, crying, stunned, and afraid. Ted looked me straight in the eyes and stated, "We can fight this. We will fight this together." He said this instinctively, for himself as much as for me. Without yet knowing or understanding what was involved, he laid the core of our belief structure: There is hope, and we will have hope. For me, my husband's words provided direction.

At the beginning of any medical trial, the role of hope is similar to that of a car engine. If the engine is cold and silent, you're going nowhere. When revved, its power introduces possibility: You can try to get to your desired destination. If all goes smoothly, you'll arrive safely and on time. If you end up taking a few wrong turns or if you're forced to take some detours, your car's engine makes it possible for you to try different routes to get to your destination or to aim for a new destination. Whether driving a car or dealing with illness, factors beyond your control will affect the ultimate path you take. Take advantage of the comfort of hope and the momentum it provides for overcoming challenges.

In the past, how much hopefulness did you bring to new problems? When problems or challenges confront you now, how hopeful do you feel at the outset?

The Power of Hope

From the time of diagnosis on, hope is the driving force behind your willingness and ability to change your situation in positive ways. Imagine that you develop an infection during your treatments. If you hope that this complication is just a temporary setback and don't conclude that it marks the beginning of the end, your hope provides the motivation needed to go through further tests and treatments. Hope not only provides energy for getting through difficult times, it also has the power to help tame your fears along the way. Hope provides a comforting counterbalance to the fear prompted by the uncertainty and discomforts of illness. For example, if you are afraid of developing progressive pain, your hope that your new medication will bring relief tames the fear, even while you are still miserable. By calming your anxiety, hope nourishes the patience, courage, and fortitude needed to go through treatment and recovery.

In addition, hope provides a powerful link between your body and your mind, and encourages you to use both, together, in your healing. The mental image of a good outcome may encourage you to eat when you're not hungry, go for a walk when you'd rather stay in bed, or report to your caregiver a symptom that you'd rather keep secret. These actions can help your body heal. And these actions can set in motion a positive feedback cycle. First, hope helps you do the right things. Then, knowing that you are improving your chances of a good outcome nourishes your sense of hope. This increased hopefulness helps you continue to do the right things, even when the challenges become greater. A positive cycle of hope makes it easier to eat, exercise, sleep, and communicate well with your health-care team.

Can hope help your physical healing *directly*? Maybe; we're not sure. As a clinician, I was stirred by the provocative idea that hope might provide some sort of mental or emotional template that helps healing in a biofeedback sort of way. We know that just as you "think the tune" of "The Star-Spangled Banner" in order to make the right notes come out of your mouth, you can learn to "think muscle relaxation." Without being able to explain exactly how you are doing it, you can learn to interrupt the subconscious tensing of your scalp muscles and relax them. So, I wondered if hope could help my patients "think" in ways that would bring pain relief, increased appetite, and other healing factors such as improved circulation to tissues in the process of repair. Scientifically, this question has barely been asked. A solid answer won't come anytime soon, since any effect of hope would be extremely complex and impossible to separate from the effects of your expectations, perceptions, will to live, and faith, let alone from the effects of your health-promoting actions.

If I can't give a definite answer, you might be wondering why I brought it up at all. One reason is that it's hard to avoid others' enthusiasm about the healing power of hope. My worry is that although the tantalizing notion that hope heals directly can be encouraging, it also can be extremely dangerous. Thinking in your head the tune to "The Star-Spangled Banner" and then hearing the right notes come out of your mouth may be complex and mysterious, *but it is a different phenomenon* than thinking in your head "kill cancer cells" or "grow new neurons" and trusting that microscopic processes that are impossible to monitor are occurring the way you want. I don't want you to fall into the guilt-ridden, joy-sapping trap of believing that if your disease doesn't respond well to your current treatment or if you suffer some complication it is because you were not hopeful enough, and that your problems are partly your own doing.

The second reason I'm bringing up this topic is that most things that can help you directly also have the potential to hurt you. An important question to consider is this: Can hope hurt you? I feel confident saying "No," nourishing hope can't hurt your recovery *as long as you get good medical care.* No evidence exists to suggest that hoping for improvement can prompt a worsening of your medical condition.

Importantly, hope opens the door to dealing with all that is beyond your control. While doing what you can to improve your situation, hope helps you let go of the many things over which you have no control. For some of you, this hope is experienced through confidence in the mysterious self-healing potential of your body. For some, it is felt through faith in God. For yet others, it is confidence that luck will be on your side. Paradoxically, letting go can give you confidence that things are under control. In giving you a sense of peace about all those things that are beyond your control, hope can help you live your life more fully each and every day, no matter what is happening medically.

Last, even though the illness resides in your body alone, your medical challenges have the effect of changing the world for those who care about you, too. Consequently, your hopefulness affects their hopefulness, which, in turn, comes back and affects your hopefulness. As my songwriting, guitar-toting rabbi, Jeffrey Leynor, sings to children, "If you drop a pebble in a pond, you can't see where all the rings have gone. [And] . . . those rings find their way back to you." Hope begets hope.

How hopeful do you feel of having a good outcome? How hopeful do you feel about being able to deal with what may lie ahead?

Know What Game You're Playing

You may find it hard to feel hopeful after you first learn that you are ill or when you develop complications or recurrences. Sometimes this discouragement is because you don't know important facts about your condition or available treatments. As a Healthy Survivor, make sure you are clear about what you are up against before deciding how hopeful you want to be. When faced with *any* challenge, you need to know the facts first. Imagine a college student, Sarah, who is invited to play a game. She's told that if she wins the game she'll get $1,000, but if she loses she must pay $2,000. Does she want to play? Sarah wisely asks to see the game before she decides. The "Game Room" is empty except for a professorial-looking gentleman sitting at a card table. A chessboard is placed in the center of the table, and all the chess pieces are lying neatly in an open velvet-lined box. Sarah's heart sinks. She was eight years old the last time she played chess. And she played against her grandfather who always let her win. Shaking her head, she declines the challenge, afraid to lose $2,000. She then returns to her dorm where her roommate is jumping up and down, squealing, "I won a thousand dollars, and I haven't played chess in years! All I needed to do was to place the pieces in the correct starting positions on the chess board."

Sarah's problem was not that she declined to play but that she turned down the opportunity before she found out the rules of the game. As a Healthy Survivor, don't give up hope before you even begin, or when you hit a bump in the road. You may be feeling discouraged because of assumptions based on myth or misinformation. Don't be like the patients who accept unnecessary pain, nausea, or fatigue because they assume these symptoms are expected and untreatable. Healthy Survivors don't give up too early. At the very least, find out what game you're playing and how to play the game before deciding how hopeful you want to be.

How well do you understand your medical situation and what you might be facing?

The Nature of Hope

Hope is not an all-or-nothing phenomenon. You can have high hope or little hope. For example, when someone gives me a flowering shrub, I usually have *little* hope of enjoying it for long because of my ineptness with plants. My children often hum a mourner's march after the gift giver is out of earshot. My hope rises if I'm told the plant is unusually hardy, or if the plant survives the first week. If I'm given a silk flower arrangement, my hope soars.

Over the years following my cancer diagnosis, my hopes as a patient waxed and waned. When I completed chemotherapy the first time, I had high hopes of enjoying a lasting remission. After the first recurrence, my hopes for a durable remission were far less. At one point, when the lymphoma returned yet again after a sixth course of treatment in as many years, I had almost no hope of a long respite from treatment. Yet now, after more than six years in remission, I am very hopeful that I'll never have lymphoma again.

Your hope is dynamic. One day, you may feel high hope. The next day, you may feel hopeless. Why the fluctuations? Your sense of hope can change depending upon how sick you feel, how much pain you have, or how tired you are. Medication effects, your innate personality, past experiences with illness, general sense of optimism, depth of faith, and how much hope your support people and health-care team project can build or weaken your sense of hopefulness, too. The next few sections will help you recognize some of the obstacles to hopefulness and think about ways to overcome them.

How strong is your sense of hope? What factors are affecting your sense of hope? Of these factors, which ones can you change?

Brain Chemistry and Hope

Hope is a feeling, so we tend to think of it as being independent of the chemistry of our cells. After all, our fancy blood tests and scanners can't detect deficiencies of hope. Hopelessness is not listed as a side effect of treatment in the thousands of pages of *The Physician's Desk Reference*

(*PDR*), and no drug has ever been designed or discovered with the sole effect of improving hopefulness.

The relationship of physical changes to thoughts and feelings is complex and mysterious. Yet, we do know that your subjective feelings such as hope and optimism are the product of chemical reactions in your brain that stimulate a particular pattern of brain cells. Presumably, it is through adverse affects on your brain chemistry that pain, fatigue, awareness of a poor prognosis, and all the other obstacles to hope mentioned earlier increase your sense of hopelessness. I'm mentioning this for three reasons: First, consider medications as a possible culprit. This is tricky since hopelessness is never listed as a side effect, but I suggest you pay particular attention to medications that are known to affect mood. Review all your elective medications (i.e., medications that could be safely discontinued) with your doctor to see if any helpful changes can be made. Second, pay attention to general health-promoting measures such as exercise, rest, and good nutrition that may help offset the negative effects of illness on the chemistry of your brain, and thus make it easier for you to experience hope. Third, I mention all this so you don't beat up on yourself if you are not feeling as hopeful as you would expect or like. Sometimes it may be difficult to feel hopeful not because you aren't trying but because your chemistry is making it hard.

Hope is a choice.

Even when discussed in physical terms, I believe that hope is unique in its resiliency. Unlike problems such as low thyroid levels, which may require intervention for improvement, you can always choose to find and nourish hope. No matter what obstacles you face and no matter what is happening, hope is a choice.

Medical Setbacks

If your condition worsens, or if your treatment appears not to be working, your sense of hope may wane. Before you let your hope slip, find out the significance of the changes in your medical condition. Are these setbacks expected or common? Do your physicians feel they are worrisome? Are they treatable? Do you have more options? You may find out that despite the current worsening you still have every reason to remain hopeful. These setbacks may be common in patients like you. Many patients suffer huge setbacks during treatment yet have a terrific outcome when it's over. Your therapy may simply need more time to work or for you to notice an improvement. If you learn that your worsening condition is a bad sign and that you are facing a more difficult situation than before, you may need to regroup in order to nourish hope.

How is your hopefulness being affected by changes in your condition?

Physical Discomforts

Physical discomfort can be an obstacle to hopefulness. When you are sick or hurting, your hopelessness may be more a reflection of your pain than of a belief that you can't or won't get better. It takes energy to maintain hope. Consequently, pain, fatigue, nausea, and other discomforts can erode your hope by draining your energy. The longer you are uncomfortable or the more miserable you feel, the harder it may be to feel hopeful or optimistic.

Even symptoms that are only a minor annoyance in the short run can wear you down when they persist for days, weeks, or longer. A colleague of mine called this the "Rubber-Band Effect." If someone snaps a small, thin rubber band against your forearm once, you might find the sensation annoying, but I doubt you'd characterize it as a debilitating pain. Yet if you kept getting snapped with little rubber bands, hour after hour, it just might drive you crazy. Recognize when physical discomfort is wearing you down, literally and figuratively.

Mary was a cancer warrior, convincingly brave and upbeat throughout the many months of chemo. One Saturday morning just after completing her treatments, a speck of dirt blew into her eye. The longer she couldn't get it out, the more upset and frazzled she became until she totally fell apart! Although a relatively minor problem, it seemed too unfair after all she'd been through. Eventually she cried it out. Tend to your physical problems, even seemingly minor ones, to help nourish your hope.

What physical problems are draining the energy you need to find and nourish hope? For each of your physical problems, what steps can you take to diminish your discomfort?

Emotional Discomforts

Feeling hopeless also may be more a reflection of your feeling emotionally distressed or depleted than a belief that you can't get better. Just as physical discomforts can siphon energy needed to maintain hope, so, too, can emotional discomforts. The longer you are under emotional strain, or the more distressed you feel, the harder it may be to feel hopeful. Tending to any emotional distress can help nourish your hope and might help you to keep your difficult moments in perspective: "I have hope; it's just hard to feel hopeful today when I feel upset (or disappointed, sad, angry, whatever.)" Talk with your health-care team about your emotions. Your physicians may be able to make adjustments in your current medications to minimize emotional side effects. Short-term treatment with antianxiety or antidepressant medications may help you feel more like yourself. Talking with family members, friends, or a counselor about your emotions may be just the support you need to work through them and regain hopefulness.

What emotional problems are draining the energy you need to find and nourish hope? For each of your emotional stressors, no matter how minor, what steps can you take to diminish your discomfort? Who can give you support?

Inaccurate Assumptions

Mistaken assumptions may decrease your ability to build hope when faced with a new medical problem. Although decisions about medical treatments should be as objective as possible, as discussed in chapter 6, preconceptions still can affect your final decision. A patient whose only image of kidney transplant is horrifying may choose to remain bedridden and dialysis dependent even though good candidates for transplant usually do well. Or, this patient may trust his doctor's advice and proceed with the surgery but, because of his frightening preconceptions, suffer excessive anxiety while awaiting the operation and afterward when any little thing goes wrong.

Any time you presume that patients in your situation never do well, you dampen or extinguish hope. The notion that recurrent disease is always the beginning of the end hampers hope and can discourage you from pursuing good treatment options when faced with a flare-up. The assumption that losing a body part or function makes you undesirable can cause you to withdraw from loved ones or hold no hope for having a passionate sexual relationship after experiencing such a loss.

If you are experiencing thoughts and feelings of hopelessness, look at them closely to see if they are based on unfounded preconceptions. Get the facts. If the facts contradict your impression, it's usually fairly easy to dismiss old ideas that dampen your hope. Seek out sound information, and talk with or read about survivors who have triumphed over similar adversity.

What preconceptions do you hold that may be hampering your sense of hopefulness?

Outdated Beliefs

Beliefs are strong convictions. Unlike assumptions and preconceptions, beliefs can be hard to shake. Try to recognize when beliefs that helped you before are now holding you back. Replace old beliefs with ones that are life enhancing in the setting of your survivorship. For example, picture someone who strongly believes that people should never leave something foreign or artificial in their bodies. Under ordinary circumstances this belief may not affect the person's life in any significant way. But if this person ever needs a coronary stent (a permanent wire that keeps open one of the arteries to the heart) or a heart-valve replacement, suddenly this long-held belief can become an obstacle to hope by making it difficult to agree to the treatment that offers the best chance of recovery. When your beliefs make it hard for you to proceed with your trusted physician's recommendations, keep in mind that conventional medical interventions are designed for people like you. Your physician would never order a test or procedure without the expectation that you would survive to reap benefits that outweigh the risks.

Take your old beliefs about illness with a grain of salt. People can't possibly know—really know—how they will feel about being seriously ill until they are patients themselves. This idea was brought home to me when I was in medical training. I learned it not only from my patients but also, in an unforgettable way, from one of my colleagues, an ICU (intensive-care unit) nurse, Kate. Both of us were young, healthy, and energetic; we became close friends while working together. In addition to seeing the run of usual medical catastrophes, we saw the effect of a particularly grueling cancer treatment on patients who were volunteers for a research study. In the fluorescent glow of the nursing station during the predawn hours, when our patients' conditions were stable and their lab results were pending, Kate and I often enjoyed exploring and sharing our philosophical beliefs about life. If anyone knew ahead of time how he or she would handle a situation, it was Kate. My nurse-friend was absolutely sure that if she ever developed a difficult-to-treat cancer like these patients, she would decline experimental treatment. She'd cared for enough patients in dire circumstances to be resolute in her conviction that she would obtain palliative care only and enjoy what she could in her remaining time.

Before I completed my medical training, that scenario was no longer a theoretical musing for my friend. She was diagnosed with a rare, aggressive, and difficult-to-treat cancer. I witnessed her transformation into a dedicated patient who willingly did exactly those things she swore she'd

decline. She underwent disfiguring surgeries, received intensive chemotherapy, and pursued risky investigational therapies with grace and hopefulness. Why the complete reversal? I suspect that her perspective as a
healthy nurse before her diagnosis led her to conclude that the pain associated with the experimental treatments was excessive and not worth it.
This belief separated her from her patients' suffering ("I'll never experience this") and freed her to devote all her energy to helping them with
expert and tender care. The cost of this belief was
that, maybe, she couldn't fully appreciate her
patients' choices and hopefulness. The unexpected turnaround in her attitude was the result
of the new perspective offered by her illness. Kate
realized that her primary value was a chance at
life, no matter how small a chance, and no matter
at how great a price. She discovered a fortitude
she never before knew she possessed.

> When you don't know the outcome, hope helps you face each new day, each new moment, and live your life.

So, what happened to Kate? Did Kate survive? Was she cured? I can tell
you that during all the months of her treatments, Kate felt she had chosen the right path for her. She was energized by the promise of cutting-
edge therapies. She felt important and proud, knowing that her youth
and vitality made her a good candidate for trial treatments, and knowing
that she was contributing something tangible, however small, to progress
in cancer care. In setting the stage for a possible recovery, she felt less
afraid and more alive than ever.

If you are bothered because I haven't yet told you if Kate made it or
not, I need to reemphasize the value of hope when dealing with illness:
When you don't know the outcome, hope helps you face each new day,
each new moment, and live your life. You can't know when you are deciding on a course of treatment, or going through treatment, if the treatment will work. You *can* know if hoping for a cure or improvement will
help you live your life today. In Kate's case, letting go of old beliefs about
hard-to-treat cancer and investigational therapies freed her to choose the
best path for her under the circumstances. Whether Kate's disease proved
resistant or responsive, and whether she ended up dying or was cured,
Kate was a Healthy Survivor because she made choices that helped her

get good care and live as fully as possible. When you are facing a new diagnosis or going through treatment and your outcome is uncertain, hope opens the door to Healthy Survivorship.

Let me stress that you don't have to choose aggressive treatment to become a Healthy Survivor. I told Kate's story to illustrate that when you are healthy you can't possibly know for sure how you would feel if you were ill. I also wanted to illustrate the value of letting go of old beliefs that keep you from Healthy Survivorship. Kate could have chosen to forgo investigational treatment and ride into the sunset just as she had predicted earlier when she was healthy. With this choice she might still harbor hopes for a miraculous recovery, but her main hopes—the hopes that would guide her everyday actions and outlook —would be to receive optimal end-of-life care and live as fully as possible in her limited remaining time. Kate could decline treatment and still be a Healthy Survivor as long as her choice was the consequence of an informed decision from her new perspective as a patient, and not because she felt trapped by her old beliefs. The hard thing for some people to grasp is that it isn't so much what path you choose that makes you a Healthy Survivor but that the path you choose is based on *informed* and *free* choices.

> A path based on informed and free choices leads to Healthy Survivorship.

Your old beliefs and decisions may or may not help you become a Healthy Survivor. Decisions made under earlier calm circumstances are not better or worse than beliefs formed under duress. On the one hand, if you happen to see your current situation just as you had expected, you would benefit from the thoughtful conclusions you drew earlier. On the other hand, your new perspective might turn your long-standing beliefs on their head as they did for Kate. You'll experience tension as your new perspective clashes with your old beliefs until you are willing to let go of your old beliefs. As a Healthy Survivor, use old beliefs that help, and let go of ones that don't.

Letting go of certain beliefs can help you nourish hope of a good out-come in nonmedical situations related to your illness, too. For instance, before your diagnosis you may have felt pity for people who had lost body parts or who used walking aids. You may have seen them as damaged goods who could never feel whole again. This conviction is just a belief, not a fact. Letting go of this narrow perspective allows you to look forward to finding new ways to feel whole after loss, even when you are thinking to yourself, "I can't see now how I can ever feel whole again, but I believe it is possible."

Another common belief shared by people who have never experienced serious illness is that survivors live every day "waiting for the other shoe to fall." This belief, if maintained, extinguishes hope of ever feeling secure and relaxed. Healthy Survivors learn that uncertainty can coexist with hopefulness for the future. Shortly into my first remission, my goal was to accept the possibility (actually, the likelihood) of recurrence while, at the same time, having confidence in my remission and putting the whole concern about recurrence at the far periphery of my life view. I believed I would get there eventually, but it took a long time before I was able to have genuine hope with acceptance. Even before you figure out how to let go of your anxiety about your future, you can nourish hope of living fully no matter what happens.

Let go of other hope-robbing beliefs such as "I can't learn anything medical. No physicians are trustworthy. The treatment is worse than the disease. People with my medical problems *never* . . . get better, feel worthy, or find happiness." An outlook shaped by old beliefs may blind you to the many possibilities and, in some cases, to the truth. Healthy Survivors abandon old beliefs that hold hope hostage in the setting of illness.

Before your illness or injury, what beliefs did you have about your medical problems or about how you would handle such problems? How are your old beliefs affecting your hopefulness?

Others' Hopelessness

The attitudes and beliefs of others can affect your sense of hope, too. If you take as gospel one doctor's declaration, "No treatments exist for your disease," you may lose all hope of recovery. So, too, you may lose all hope when your doctor suggests that you'd do best to accept that you will never be able to improve your energy, get pregnant, or overcome the particular medical challenge you are facing. Feeling hopeless, you probably would not pursue second opinions or trials of therapies that other reputable physicians believe might give you a real chance. It is not just the medical experts who can dampen your belief in your ability to improve your outcome. If your family and friends express despair (verbally or nonverbally), you may find it harder to maintain your own sense of hopefulness, even if you want to.

Genuine hope arises from within you, not from some external source. If you want to feel hopeful, try to see others' attitude of hopelessness as *their* problem, not yours. Separate your beliefs from those of people who express pessimism and hopelessness despite the possibility of improvement. When you can, let people know when they are dragging you down. If they can't see why you still have hope, and if they insist on sharing their hopelessness, tactfully tell them to keep their feelings to themselves when they are with you. Avoid them if you must in order to hold on to your hope. You have a right to be hopeful.

How are your family and friends helping your hopefulness?
How are they hurting it?

Other Patients' Past Medical Disasters

Hearing or reading descriptions of others' past medical disasters unleashes raw emotions and hampers hope. The health trials of famous people become part of our communal culture, and their personal illnesses help define specific maladies. Ovarian cancer is called "Gilda's Disease," in reference to the comedienne Gilda Radner, who was treated for this disease at a young age. What is the first thing a woman thinks after being diagnosed with ovarian cancer? Gilda *died*.

The illnesses of your friends, family, and neighbors also influence your preconceptions and beliefs, often in profound ways. Let's say your neighbor developed early heart disease with a good prognosis yet died of an unexpected heart attack. Your personal knowledge of this unusual and sad scenario may dampen your faith in all conventional cardiac treatments. Certainly, it can shake your confidence if, later, you are diagnosed with a similar heart condition. Despite your own excellent prognosis, you may find it difficult to feel hopeful because of your intimate knowledge of the real, though small, possibility of a poor outcome.

Try to recognize when your knowledge of others' past problems is affecting your hopefulness. Take steps in your own mind to unlink your medical situation from everyone else's. Separating yourself may be easy. For example, when someone not so tactfully said to me, "Oh, you have the same disease that killed Jackie Kennedy," I wasn't bothered at all because I knew that Kennedy's type of non-Hodgkin's was a different lymphoma than mine. Separating yourself may be hard. A friend's husband was diagnosed with the same type of leukemia that had taken the life of his younger brother a few years earlier. At first, my friend's husband refused all treatment, saying "We know the outcome. I want to let it happen fast and spare my family prolonged suffering so they can move on with their lives." The vivid memories of his brother's illness made it hard for him to find any hope for himself. Counselors and family members acknowledged that he and his brother were genetically more similar than strangers. But, just as you can flip a coin in seemingly the exact same way and get heads one time and tails another, he still could hope that he would land on the good side of the statistics even though his brother hadn't. They encouraged him to focus on the many ways he and his brother were indisputably different, such as their heights, weights, and temperaments. Importantly, his doctors now had access to new treatments, treatments that might have cured his brother had they been available when he was ill. My friend's husband realized that he was a unique individual and chose, with hope, to get treated.

When what you know about other patients makes it hard for you to feel hopeful about yourself, remember that these stories and memories tell you about other people, not about you. Every situation is unique. Don't tack on someone else's ending to your story. *Your* story will unfold as you live it, and not before!

Whom do you know who has suffered from conditions similar to yours? How can you separate from these memories?

Others' Current Medical Problems

A special challenge to hope is your knowledge of another patient's current misfortune. The death of *Superman* actor Christopher Reeve rocked the hope of thousands of patients with chronic medical problems, especially the hope shared by people with spinal-cord injuries. From all media reports, Mr. Reeve had everything going for him. He vowed in inspiring interviews that he would walk again, one day. His confidence was contagious given his access to the highest-tech medical care, his political connections and savvy, the constant loving support he received from family, friends, and millions of fans, and his extraordinary courage and will to live. If anyone could do it, it was Reeve. Over the nine years since his accident, reports of his path-breaking incremental recoveries—increased sensation and an ability to wiggle a finger—fueled everyone's hope. His untimely death due to a common (and feared) complication of quadriplegia reminds everyone of the limits of the body, mind, and spirit when faced with overwhelming illness.

Even if your disease is responding nicely to current therapy or you are enjoying a remission, learning that things aren't going well for someone else may shake your hope, especially if that someone is going through similar medical challenges. In addition to the fact that this patient *does* have access to the same cutting-edge medicine as you, it may be hard because the real-time drama taps into your emotions in a way that past events don't. It may break through to your rational understanding of the bad outcomes that are possible for you. Yet another potential reason for the clout of these stories is empathy: You can imagine only too well what it is like to get bad news. If this could happen to her, it could happen to you. Last, even if you are not too concerned about yourself, your empathy for the particular patient stirs general feelings such as sadness, anger, fear, and vulnerability.

Try to be sensitive to how stories about other patients might be affecting you. Make an effort to distance yourself by focusing on specific differences between you and that patient. Separate your feelings of empathy for the other person from stirred-up feelings about you. If you can, turn your anxiety into heightened appreciation for how well you are doing.

How is your case special? What factors might give you an advantage over other patients in your situation?

Flexibility

An ability to adapt gracefully to the ups and downs of life is touted as a key element to longevity. Given the many changes and challenges that accompany living with illness, it seems logical that flexibility would be a valuable trait for survivors. Besides helping you save energy while adjusting to new situations, being flexible helps you nourish hope. Everyone is flexible to one degree or another. To give you a silly example, I won't buy gourmet bottled water from the grocery store because it is so pricey. However, when my family goes to volleyball tournaments, I'm willing to shell out top dollar for a brand of bottled water that is usually inexpensive. Especially when we are at tournaments in gyms with no other access to water, sticking rigidly to arbitrary budget rules would take away any hope of satisfying my thirst.

Your flexibility can affect your care. Personal modesty may cause you to be unwilling to expose private body parts. If your reserve keeps you from sharing important information about your condition with your health-care team, you may lose hope of obtaining optimal care. Being flexible—shedding your usual modesty—can help you. You may find writing down your concern easier than speaking out loud. Just know that you need to find a way—your way—of communicating. As another example, a certain amount of self-sufficiency helps you function well at work and at home. After a diagnosis, an unwillingness to let go of any independence while you are receiving energy-draining treatments could backfire on you. Overextending yourself could lead to exhaustion or medical setbacks that dampen your hope of getting through treatment. Illness provides opportunities to practice flexibility. A willingness to let go of old ways that are no longer adaptive may help you regain some control over your situation. Try to let go of personal rules and guidelines that worked well before but hold you back now.

How flexible are you? What long-standing thoughts, beliefs, and approaches might be holding you back? How can you let go of old ways that are no longer helping you?

Multiply Hopes

"Don't put all your eggs in one basket" is an aphorism that warns against the danger of having only one hope. An athlete whose one and only dream is to hear his national anthem as he receives an Olympic gold medal may see himself as a failure if he doesn't snatch one, even if he performs his personal best and wins an Olympic silver. Patients may be tempted to invest in a single hope such as cure. Unless their disease is cured with surgery alone, cure is a goal that, at best, is rewarded only after weeks or months of treatments, during which time delays or setbacks can erode hope. Even if everything goes smoothly, a single long-term goal may not provide you the motivation needed on a daily basis to get through. If cure is your only goal, you might have to wait years to feel satisfied. In general, grand goals are fine as long as they are not your only goals.

The more things you hope for, the more hope you may have. Nourishing your hope for a smaller achievement doesn't diminish your hope for a grander goal any more than loving one child diminishes your love for another. If anything, hope feeds hope. Having hope of getting through today's treatment, and this week's treatment, and this month's treatments may help you nourish your hopes of completing all

If hopes are dashed, shift your focus to hopes that remain and create new hopes.

your treatments and achieving remission. Let's say your ultimate hope is to return to work. You may feel encouraged every day by picturing yourself back at your office, thus nourishing your hope for this end. Day in and day out, your smaller hopes—such as the hope of getting off intravenous medicines, being discharged from the hospital, and regaining mobility—can strengthen your overall hope of becoming well enough to work. Nurturing a variety of hopes increases the chance of seeing at least some of your hopes come to fruition. The emotional lift of small successes feels good and nourishes optimism. Should one particular hope be dashed, you can soften your disappointment by shifting your focus to your hopes that remain and by creating new hopes.

What are your various hopes about your physical condition? What are your hopes about things other than your physical well-being? Make a list of everything you hope for today. Make a new list to see you through difficult times.

Language

Language is powerful. Of all the factors that affect your sense of hope, language is comparatively easy to manipulate to your advantage. For instance, a term commonly used to describe a patient is *victim*. Its negative connotations of helplessness and hopelessness are obvious. In contrast, *survivors* continue on despite challenge or threat. I am always a cancer survivor, sometimes a cancer patient, but never a cancer victim. Cancer victims and cancer survivors are people in the same situation with different frames of mind.

Victims and survivors are people in the same situation with different frames of mind.

Language is powerful. I've had repeated recurrences not because, as oncologists say, "I failed my treatments," but because my treatments failed me. My type of lymphoma is not incurable, as decreed by the textbooks. Rather, it is one of the types of lymphoma for which scientists are still looking for a cure. Wordplay is not trivial mental gymnastics; it is one of the forces that shape patients' perceptions of reality. Listen to yourself when talking with others or to yourself in your head. If your language reveals underlying feelings such as fear or anger, find a safe place to explore these feelings so that you can overcome obstacles to hope. In the meantime, use hopeful language. It will help you feel better. You have a right to encourage others to use hopeful language, too. (See appendix II.)

Do you think of yourself as a victim or a survivor? How hopeful is your language when talking about your situation?

Measuring Triumph

Every week I hear or read in the obituaries about someone who "lost" his or her long (or brave) battle with some illness. Equating physical death with failure implies that every single human being is a failure. Triumph over illness is measured by *how* one lives, not how long. A patient who lives six months while receiving excellent medical care and who is physically comfortable and able to appreciate the company of friends and family has triumphed. A patient who spends forty years in complete remission, feeling bitter about his or her bout of illness or withdrawn from society due to lost self-esteem, has succumbed. What matters most is not when you die or what you die from but what you live for in whatever time you have.

> Triumph over illness is measured by *how* you live, not how long.

How do you measure triumph over illness?

Positive Attitude

What role does a positive attitude play in your recovery? Can a positive attitude cure you without the use of conventional therapies? How is a positive attitude related to optimism and hope? What is a positive attitude, anyway? These are important questions because so many people talk about the over-riding role of a positive attitude in healing. Unfortunately, people confuse *positive attitude* with *sustained optimism* or *hopefulness*. To complicate matters, many people believe that an unwavering expectation or hope of doing well will help them get well. The problem is that such a belief can create undue stress and may be harmful. It doesn't seem reasonable for me to expect to feel optimistic when I first learn bad news about my condition.

> A positive attitude is one that helps you get good care and live as fully as possible.

So, what is a positive attitude? For Healthy Survivors, a positive attitude is an attitude that helps you get good care and live as fully as possible. Since your circumstances are always changing, and since you are an individual, what constitutes a positive attitude is fluid and unique to you. My positive attitude is based on optimism and hopefulness yet allows for periods of pessimism and hopelessness.

What constitutes a positive attitude for you?

Optimism and Hope

Optimism and hopefulness arise because of uncertainty. When the outcome is assured, you don't need optimism or hope. You wouldn't say, "I'm optimistic (or hopeful) that gravity will continue to hold me on the ground." So, too, if your complete recovery were assured, optimism and hope would be irrelevant because you would know the outcome. But for those of you for whom a cure is unlikely with current treatment, optimism and hope play major roles in helping you handle the uncertainty and unpredictability of living with chronic illness.

> *Optimism: the tendency to expect a favorable outcome.*
> *Hope: the belief that it is possible to have a favorable outcome.*

Optimism is not the same as hope. Your level of optimism reflects your *expectations* regarding the desired outcome. In contrast, the strength of your hopefulness reflects your *belief in the possibility* of the desired outcome. Optimism is a state of mind. Hopefulness is a state of heart. Optimism and hopefulness may go hand in hand. Let's say you have painful gallstones. If you are otherwise healthy, your surgeon might explain that you are in a high-success category for both getting through surgery and being cured of your pain. Since a perfect outcome can't be guaranteed, your optimism and hope are brought into play. In this particular case, you would have every reason to be very optimistic (to expect a good outcome) *and* hopeful (to believe in the possibility of your having a good outcome).

Your sense of optimism can be off-kilter with your sense of hope, too. Let's say that your illness is causing you to experience pain that has not been relieved by first- and second-line analgesics (pain medications). When your physician recommends a third-line drug that works in 10 percent of patients, you may understand and believe it is possible for you to obtain relief. You have hope. Yet, at the same time, you may be pessimistic and expect the medications to fail. In this same situation, other patients might be both optimistic and hopeful. Namely, they truly expect to be that one in ten whose pain goes away.

How much optimism or hope should you have? Only you can answer that because it depends on your situation, and on you. You can use both optimism and hope in ways that help you get good medical care and live as fully as possible. In each situation you face, you have to find a unique balance of optimism and hope that works best for you.

As a Healthy Survivor, try to find levels of optimism and hope that

- are in touch with the facts of your condition;
- feel true and comfortable;
- help you accept your current condition;
- help you look to the future with hopefulness, be it hopefulness for recovery, pain relief, or meaningful connection with loved ones;
- motivate you to do the right things to get better, when improvement is possible;
- connect you with those you love and care about.

How optimistic do you feel? How hopeful do you feel? Do you feel you have the right balance of the two?

Optimism and Healing

An expectation of doing well may help indirectly by giving you the energy and discipline needed to find out about treatment options, make wise decisions, and then comply with treatments, eat well, get in condition, sleep more restfully, and feel less stressed. Researchers are exploring the possibility that genuine optimism—the honest expectation of doing well—may cause physical changes in your body that contribute directly to your healing in much the same way proposed for hope earlier in this chapter. If optimism helps healing directly to some degree, it is most helpful in the setting of optimal treatments. And, optimism can't hurt you as long as you are getting good medical care.

The trap is to think that maintaining an attitude of unwavering optimism can effect a cure. The notion that your mind can *control* your physical healing is engaging and popular but has never been proven. Even the most optimistic state of mind and heart cannot guarantee you a good medical outcome. Knowing this fact liberates you to be yourself and not feel guilty or like a failure should you develop complications or progressive disease. You have enough genuine concerns; you don't need to feel guilty about your condition, too. Be kind to yourself. The best you can do is the best you can do.

How would you rate your overall level of optimism?

Healthy Optimism

Optimism can lead you *to* or *away from* Healthy Survivorship. On the one hand, optimism helps you when it leads you to be vigilant about your checkups ("I expect to do fine because my physicians and I are keeping close tabs on my progress"). On the other hand, optimism can be problematic when it leads you to abandon follow-up exams ("I expect to do fine, so I don't need my physicians to keep tabs on me"). Optimism is comforting when it encourages patience ("I can wait however long it takes to feel better because I expect the end result to be

When is your optimism helping you? When is it hurting you?

worth it"). Or, optimism is anxiety provoking when it leads to impatience ("I should feel better right now!"). You may be inspired by optimism ("Telling myself I'm going to do well makes it easier to go through treatment"). Or, you may tire of trying to maintain a sense of optimism, especially when it forces you to act differently than how you really feel at the moment ("I'm exhausted trying to be upbeat for everyone all the time!"). When an optimistic attitude helps you heal, it nourishes hope. When optimism keeps you from acting effectively, it hurts your chance for recovery and, thereby, encourages false hope. Use healthy optimism to help you obtain sound knowledge, find and nourish hope, and act effectively.

Optimism in Patients with Terminal Disease

What about patients who remain steadfastly optimistic about recovery despite relentless deterioration in their medical condition? Is this optimism good or bad? It depends. A belief that attitude is an all-powerful factor in healing may lead some patients to try to remain fiercely optimistic no matter what is happening. When this optimism is genuine, these people truly anticipate a miraculous rescue and find satisfaction and meaning in daily life with this outlook. For others, this show of optimism belies all the doubts they harbor but feel obligated to hide, even from themselves, leading to loneliness and emotional misery.

If you want to feel more optimistic, you can work toward having a genuine expectation of doing well no matter what the statistical odds. You can look for a doctor who shares your optimism, even if not to the same degree, and who shares your willingness to try another treatment that offers even a sliver of hope. You can ask friends and relatives to express only optimism, at least when they are with you.

When the end is near, unfounded optimism can exact a price. Avoiding all thought and discussion of the possibility of death can have the unintended consequence of causing you to sacrifice meaningful conversations of closure with loved ones. In your time remaining, your interaction with others is characterized by superficiality rather than a full and deep mining of your relationship. For other patients, accepting that death is imminent frees them to have those conversations or final experiences that give meaning and closure for themselves and their loved ones. The price of this shaping of one's legacy is the immediate pain of losing hope, not necessarily all hope, but at least some hope for at least a short while. And this expressed acceptance of a poor outcome may precipitate conflict with family members and friends who are not ready to give up hope. Always keep in mind that expecting to die doesn't obligate you to die. If after preparing for your funeral, giving away your favorite jewelry, and saying all your "good-byes" you make an amazing recovery, you don't have to jump off a cliff. You can say "Hello! Cancel the funeral," then ask for your jewelry back and get on with your life.

A friend of mine showed me the value of accepting impending death and, at the same time, fighting it. After many rounds of aggressive treatment, and after recovering from a complication that had her lingering in the intensive-care unit near death for a couple of weeks, she learned that her most recent scans revealed advanced, probably treatment-resistant disease. She chose to say her good-byes and prepare her daughter to continue on after her death, accepting that her remaining time was likely very limited. Yet she also continued to receive investigational treatments in clinical trials and, when trials were not available, petitioned to receive promising drugs under compassionate-use guidelines. Her actions spoke volumes: Acceptance doesn't obligate you to give up hope. I can't help wondering if her combination of peacefulness and feistiness, of acceptance and hopefulness, helped the last-ditch treatments work well enough to give her a series of temporary reprieves. Her life after saying her first good-byes was measured in years, not months. During those years, she lived life with a fullness of purpose and spirit.

Tempered optimism can be life enhancing in the setting of terminal illness. But for some patients, unwavering optimism is their path to a good death, and it helps when those caring for this patient respect this choice. You have to find your own balance. Gauge the facts about the possibilities for people in your situation, and adopt a level of optimism that leads you to your best quality of life.

What level of optimism helps you get good care? What level of optimism helps you feel best on a day-to-day basis?

Optimism and Your Physicians

Your physicians have a unique role in your care, as well as obligations when sharing their expectations about your course or outcome. Your doctors provide the interface between scientific knowledge about *you* and scientific knowledge about *your illness based on populations of people*. They can provide sound information about what is happening right now and offer a projection based on available data about other patients. Physicians who care deeply and who want you to do well serve you best by being honest about their expectations. Make sure that your physician's level of optimism about your situation is only one factor of many that helps shape your own level of optimism. Remember: Expectations are not predictions. No human being can *predict* your future. And, your physicians' *expectations* based on scientific information and personal experience do not reflect their *hopes* or *desires*.

When asked about the prognosis of patients with terminal disease, I would discuss what to expect and how to prepare for the likely events. In conclusion, I shared my hopes. "Sometimes things happen in medicine that we don't understand. I want you to get better. I am prepared for the likely outcome and hoping for a good outcome for you. I'll be here for you whatever happens."

What does your health-care team hope for you?

Learned Optimism

Everyday situations can unexpectedly reveal underlying pessimism or smoldering fears, as well as offer opportunities to teach you optimism. As a regular subscriber to the prestigious *New England Journal of Medicine* when I was practicing medicine, I'd never hesitated to take advantage of the cost savings of renewing it for three years at a time. While recovering from my first round of chemotherapy and trying to be hopeful about my future, the little white renewal card arrived in the mail, and the sight of it paralyzed me. Should I shell out the cash and renew it for three years, as usual, or renew it for one year this time, if at all? If I don't renew, am I sending my body a "die" message? My angst over a stupid journal renewal notice exposed how insecure I felt about my health. Writing a check and sending it together with my renewal form offered me an opportunity to build hope and optimism about my future.

That same summer, after almost thirteen years of marriage, Ted and I decided to buy a new bed. Ours was getting soft and lumpy, and we worried that it might be slowing down the recovery of the nerve in my leg that had been damaged earlier by a tumor pressing on it. At the local mall, Ted enthusiastically lay down on one mattress after another while I wandered aimlessly among the sheetless beds. We didn't buy a bed that evening. Back at home, Ted asked what was wrong, and I surprised even myself when I answered, "I don't want to buy my deathbed. I don't want to buy a bed you might sleep in without me one day." In the context of buying a mattress, my suppressed waves of fear and pessimism surfaced. Ted responded with blended tenderness and firmness: "Wendy, buying a bed will have no impact on your cancer. We need a new bed, a really good one so we can sleep better now. Let's get one with an extended warranty because I'm planning on sleeping in it—with you!—for a long time." That snapped me out of my pessimism. In no way would I let my negativity keep us from dealing with the real, practical, immediate problem. Buying a top-of-the-line, double-sided, pillow-top mattress with a twenty-five-year warranty became my way of shaking my fist at my fears and turning pessimism into optimism. Ever since, Ted periodically pats our bed and winks at me. "Mighty comfortable bed we have!"

Appearing Optimistic While Feeling Pessimistic

Appearing optimistic is not the same as *being* optimistic. Like most things about survivorship, trying to appear optimistic when you are feeling down can be good or bad for you at any particular time. A charade of optimism may cause internal stress, confusion, anger, or helplessness that outweighs any benefits. Without a place to share or work through your pessimism, feigned optimism can be draining and make you feel *less* hopeful instead of more so.

Is it helping you or hurting you to appear optimistic right now?

Alternatively, walking the walk and talking the talk of optimism can be a conscious strategy. Lots of people have found that acting up when they're down changes their outlook and how they feel in positive ways. Certainly, it changes how others relate to them, and that can begin a positive feedback cycle, too. Don't worry about being dishonest if you are trying to appear more optimistic than you really are feeling. If it makes you feel better in any way, pretending to be optimistic may lay seeds of genuine optimism that help you.

Pessimists and Hope

What's wrong with pessimism? Pessimism can be an advantage for some people in certain situations. Holding on to pessimism gives some people the comfort of familiarity and the confidence of feeling in control of their attitude. One man in my support group was a curmudgeon, constantly complaining and as pessimistic as they come. In a self-deprecating way, he laughed at his gloomy nature and invited others to, also. Instead of feeling forced to act in a way he didn't feel, and a way that would have felt uncomfortably unnatural, he used his pessimism in helpful ways.

When dealing with medical problems, the danger is that a negative outlook may pull you down. If your prognosis is good with effective treatments, pessimism may keep you from pursuing measures that can help you. Expecting things to go badly may keep you from taking charge of factors that are under your control for your healing. You may see no point in getting second opinions or adjusting your diet, sleep, or exercise regimens. Since you don't expect to get well, you may subconsciously be lax about your medical therapies, too. You may not be inclined to put in the effort needed to adjust to the changes and losses. In other words, pessimism can trigger behaviors that sabotage your healing.

Your blue moods may alienate you from people who care about you, too. When physicians and therapists are giving you their best efforts but sense that you don't expect benefit, or that you aren't doing your part, they may be put off. Implied or openly expressed pessimism communicates to others "You're wasting your time since I'm not going to do well, anyway." I'd like to think that every professional gives his or her best effort to every single patient irrespective of their attitude, and that your loved ones will hang in there with you no matter what. Realistically speaking, some of your physicians, nurses, family, or friends may find it hard to deal with your pessimism and its implied lack of respect for their efforts.

> Don't let pessimism about tomorrow steal joy you could have today.

Pessimism can steal good times. Vickie is a patient who awoke every morning thinking "Today might be the day it comes back." Having completed treatment for a disease with a high rate of recurrence, she withdrew from friends and activities, convinced she'd soon be sick again. After seven years of living like a hermit, she awoke one morning to the terrible realization "I've been healthy all this time, and I missed it."

As explained in earlier sections, pessimism does not determine outcome. Many crotchety patients with pessimistic outlooks do fabulously well throughout their treatments and recoveries. For some, it is a variation of magical thinking that helps them cope. Like the straight-"A" student who announces before every single exam "I'm going to fail!" these patients predict that they will do badly while, in their hearts, they expect a good outcome. This is not real pessimism but a negative front. For others, the pessimism is genuine. Yet, when they make wise decisions with their physicians and comply with treatments, they surprise themselves and do well.

When you express pessimism, is it helping you or hurting you?

Using Your Mind to Help Your Heart Find Hope

It's not a big problem if hopelessness is your initial reaction or a momentary state. It's when hopelessness becomes your permanent frame of reference and keeps you from acting effectively that it can prevent Healthy Survivorship. In general, it is easier to change your *thoughts* about the hopefulness of your situation than to change your *feelings* of hope, and you can use the strength of your rational mind to reshape your emotional outlook. For instance, if the statistics indicate that 60 percent of patients in your situation recover, you may feel defeated. The first step toward Healthy Hope is acknowledging that more than half of the patients like you are expected to have a good outcome. Now, ask yourself if you believe—in a cold, statistical sort of way—if it is possible for *you* to be one of the 60 percent who do well. If you do (and surely you do), then you can use your rational thoughts to reshape your feelings. You can use the indisputable fact that you have a reasonable chance of doing well to start building genuine feelings of hopefulness, no matter how pessimistic you are by nature. Look for a point of optimism you can accept on a rational level, and then teach yourself to *feel* what you *know*.

*Can you think of times when you can use your knowledge of
possible good outcomes to help you feel more optimistic?*

Statistics and Hope

Statistics can build or weaken your hope, depending on how you use them. Statistics—analyzed numerical data on past populations of patients—affected my sense of hope soon after my first diagnosis. On the one hand, the statistics were comforting because my type of lymphoma was classified as a slow-growing cancer. Statistically speaking, my life was not in imminent danger. On the other hand, state-of-the-art conventional lymphoma therapies offered the possibility of cure only for the rapidly advancing types. So, statistically speaking, patients like me with indolent lymphomas were never cured. As discussed in chapter 5, I needed to understand the strengths and limits of statistics for them to nourish my hope.

Good statistics are hopeful, so hold on to their message when you have solid reason to expect a good outcome. But even upsetting statistics can help nourish your hope. When you use statistics to help you make wise treatment decisions with your doctors, the statistics are helping you and your doctors stack the odds in your favor, giving you more reason to feel hopeful. Then, once treatment begins, determine if statistics are helping you now. You may find the inspiration needed to contend with unpleasant treatments when you remind yourself that your statistics *are best* with your chosen treatment. Even the grimmest statistics can help if they pique your fighting spirit and cause you to shout, "I'll show everybody. I'll be the exception to the rule!"

If you feel oppressed by bad statistics, forget about them! Statistics are not the same as your reality, now or ever. Nobody on earth can *foresee* how you will do, even if using the most detailed statistics, sophisticated tests and scans, plentiful anecdotes, or powerful premonitions. Unless you have zero chance of improvement, you have reason for hope. In the prologue to this book, I shared the story of William at bat. It was the bottom of the last inning, and the score was tied. Two kids were on base, and

seven-year-old Will came up to the plate. On the first pitch, Will swung—
whoosh—six inches above the ball. On the next pitch he swung and
whiffed it again, this time six inches *below* the ball. On average, he got a
hit! Of course, the ball was in the catcher's glove and it was "Strike two."
Just as important as illustrating the gap between statistical outcome and
reality, this story highlights the concept of hope. There is always hope.

How are you using your statistics to nourish hope?

Bumblebees of Hope

Well-documented patient stories begin "Against all odds . . . ," or "Much
to everyone's surprise . . . ," or "Despite the doctors' predictions. . . ."
Remarkable, unexpected, and unexplained recoveries and reprieves occur
every day. Sometimes, even when doctors think the chance is zero, they turn
out to be wrong. Until we unravel the remaining mysteries of illness and
healing, and as long as you are alive, your chance for recovery is not zero.
The uncertainty surrounding your situation gives you reason to be hopeful.

When I was in medical practice, I saw patients who by all medical
indicators should have done poorly. I called them my "bumblebee
patients." Somewhere I'd heard that, according to the general laws of
physics, the bumblebee's body weight is too great for its wing size to
accommodate flying. Bumblebees don't know that, so they fly! My bumblebee patients had diseases or chest X rays or blood-test results that
appeared incompatible with functional life. Yet they kept coming for
checkups, telling me about their adventures or responsibilities that did
not leave time for being sick, or about their excitement about a forthcoming grandchild or graduation. As a Healthy Survivor, remember the
bumblebee. Recoveries happen that we can't explain.

The bumblebee metaphor is instructive because the ability of bumblebees to fly does not defy the general laws of physics. Rather, further
advances in our understanding of flight physics were needed before scientists could explain the phenomenon of bumblebee flight. So, too,

patients' unexpected and inexplicable recoveries are just that: unexplained. Scientific explanations are forthcoming; we must await further advances in science and technology before researchers can explain them in terms we understand. Once a patient's surprising recovery is understood, researchers will use the insights to develop treatments that will make the unexpected and inexplicable expected and understandable and reproducible.

Especially when you are first diagnosed, it helps to nourish hope for recovery no matter how lopsided the statistics. You have as good a chance of responding as anyone else in your risk group. Today's survivors of devastating disease or illness—and there are millions of them—are living proof of the notion that there is always hope. Somebody lands on the good side of the statistics; it might as well be you.

Hopeful Stories

Stories can offer the *feeling* of hope. You may find it helpful to read books and articles by survivors of unfavorable odds. Talking with real, live people who landed on the good side of bad statistics can help nourish your hope that you, too, will do well. My long ordeal with cancer recurrences has given me opportunities to experience the effects of statistics and others' stories on my sense of hopefulness. After my lymphoma recurred a second time, I decided to enter a clinical trial of an experimental treatment. When I was first given the treatment, I was the fifteenth person ever to receive it, so nobody knew if it would work at all, let alone how long it would work. Living in the uncharted territory of a treatment with no statistics, I felt free to be hopeful that it would put my cancer into a complete remission for a long, long time. The new therapy caused a significant reduction in my tumor and put my cancer into a partial remission that lasted about eight months. After the next course of the same treatment, this time given in a higher dose, my cancer went into a complete remission that lasted about ten months. By the time I received a fourth round of the antibody treatment, a few statistics from the earlier trials had just become available, showing an average duration of effect that matched my experience: ten months. Unlike when I had no statistics to shape my expectations, I now had a data point—ten months—that made it harder for me to feel hopeful about getting a lasting remission from the drug. I knew it was still possible, but I found it harder to believe with my heart what I believed in my head. It was fine to let statistics change my *expectations;* they didn't have to dampen my *hope.*

About that time, I met a woman at a conference who had received the same treatment as I. She'd received it four years earlier when she had advanced disease, and her cancer went into a complete remission and stayed there. For me, talking to someone who was living proof of what was possible helped me feel more hopeful that my own remission might last for years. Expectation is a state of mind; hope is a state of heart. Putting a real name and a face to the possibility of long-term success helped me have hope. As it turns out, despite three episodes of response lasting eight to ten months, and despite the statistics suggesting I should expect a similar experience, the fourth round of treatment I received gave me a lasting remission, one that continues over six years later.

What stories can help you nourish hope?

Research and Hope

Clinical trials are tests of new therapies on people. They offer hope to everyone. Patients who participate in clinical trials nourish hope because trials are established only when earlier studies suggest the treatment under investigation will work. And, reality-based hope is stronger than that based solely on wishful thinking. Ongoing research also gives hope to those of you who are not participating in a clinical trial. How? With research, you can hope that if your standard treatments don't cure you, they will help you live long enough to benefit from better remedies that come along. That is exactly what happened to me. The first rounds of chemotherapy, radiation therapy, and interferon therapy did not cure my lymphoma. They didn't even provide lasting remissions. What they did do was control my disease long enough for me to benefit from a new chemotherapy that first became available five years after my original diagnosis, as well as to benefit long-term from the less toxic and equally effective (for me) antibody therapy that was FDA approved seven years after my original diagnosis. If I end up needing more treatment in the future, and if the newer treatments I've already received stop working for me, an even newer and better treatment may be available. As a Healthy Survivor, take comfort in the hope offered by research.

Nourishing Hope

Hope can shrivel away if not nourished, sometimes without your even realizing it. Just as you need to refill your gas tank regularly when driving long distances, you need to nourish your hope while living with the challenges of illness. During my first round of chemotherapy, my hopes were solid. With so many things going for me, I referred to myself as "the princess with cancer." Young and otherwise healthy, I had sophisticated medical knowledge that enabled me to be an expert patient as I received state-of-the art intensive therapy from a caring medical team. My husband adored me. My three young children needed me. I had an ever-deepening spiritual faith. Instinctively and deeply, I had hope of surviving, hope of getting through treatment, and hope of helping my children through it all.

Over the years of contending with my recurrent lymphoma, my hopes for cure and long life were tested over and over again. As I embarked on each course of treatment, friends and family would say to me, "I hope this treatment is the one that cures you." In 1991 and 1992, and, maybe, in 1993, I'd answer, "I hope so, too." I don't know exactly when my answer shifted, but after a while I found myself answering, "Oh, I can be happy and feel fulfilled even if I need to be treated every year." In the spring of 1995, soon after starting a new course of chemotherapy, one friend heard the resignation in that reply and blurted out, "Well, I hope this treatment gets rid of the cancer forever!"

Somewhere between the fifth and sixth courses of treatment, without my even realizing it, my hopes for cure and for long life had slipped away. I was so determined to be grateful for whatever life I had that I'd stopped hoping so that I wouldn't feel disappointed or angry whenever scans revealed progressive or new disease. With that realization, I renewed my hope and have been nourishing it actively ever since. Pay attention to your sense of hope the way you'd watch your weight or level of conditioning, so you can nourish your hope throughout treatment and recovery.

How strong is your hope for your future compared to last week? Last month? Last year?

Lost Hope

One obstacle to hopefulness is fear of being disappointed or being wrong. If you've been disappointed in the past, either related to your current medical problems or with other important situations in your life, you may be reluctant to feel hopeful. Withholding hope may seem the logical way to protect yourself from future disappointment. Supposedly, if you aren't hopeful and then things go badly, you'll feel better than if you'd been hopeful all along. In my case, this certainly isn't true. Whenever I learned that my cancer had progressed or recurred, I experienced enough fear and sadness to overwhelm any satisfaction I might have felt for being right had I predicted it.

Choosing hopelessness is an approach beset with problems. Lack of hope may keep you from making wise treatment decisions because you're focusing on the downsides of each option. Hopelessness may keep you from feeling confident about your treatment decisions and may make it harder to deal with any discomforts, inconveniences, and setbacks that arise during treatment. Expecting the worst, you might notice and focus on insignificant side effects and problems, or misinterpret side effects or minor complications as evidence of progressive disease. Think about all of the elements of hope before deciding how hopeful you want to be. Be true to yourself about what helps. Throughout your survivorship, stay in touch with your sense of hope. If hope starts to slip away, take steps to find and nourish the hope that helps you do what you need to do to live most fully.

How often do you do a "hope" check? What are you doing to help nourish your hope over the long haul?

Hopeful Acceptance

When you are not expected to get well, you don't have to choose between (1) accepting that your condition will likely continue to decline and (2) hoping that things will get better. You can both accept that your medical condition is deteriorating, or that the chance for improvement is small, yet at the same time have genuine hope for improvement. For many years now, I've understood and accepted that no known cures have been available for my type of cancer. I now accept that I will most likely die of my lymphoma or a treatment- or disease-related complication, such as infection. At the same time, I have genuine hope for cure and long life. A magazine story that ran soon after the 1995 accident that paralyzed actor Christopher Reeve described this paradox when they quoted him as saying he both accepted his disability and chose to fight it. The balance between hope and acceptance seesaws depending on your

Negative thoughts and feelings can coexist with a deep faith in a complete recovery.

realities at the moment. As the facts grow grimmer, hope gets dimmer. But, like one or two stars peeking through the clouds on a moonless night, even a ray of hope brings comforting light to the gloom. Over the years, I've had my share of pessimistic thoughts and times of hopelessness. Negative thoughts or dreams don't diminish overall solid hope unless you dwell on them or interpret them to mean that your hope is weak. Having moments or hours of hopelessness and fears and anxieties about a poor outcome means you are human, not despairing. When you know that negative thoughts and feelings can coexist with a deep faith in a complete recovery, you tame your fears and anxieties, avoid despair, and nourish hope.

Prepare for the Worst

You may wonder (or your family and friends may wonder) if being hopeful in the face of a poor prognosis isn't hope but, rather, a form of denial. For most people, denial is seen as a bad thing because it keeps you from dealing with reality. When the outlook is grim, denial can keep you from completing a living will or saying and doing things you would if magically you knew the exact limits of your time.

Preparing for the worst does not necessarily diminish your hope. Paradoxically, feeling ready for the worst may free you to have hope. I remember one woman who was diagnosed with a brain tumor. She was pessimistic about her future, so prepared her will, gave away many belongings, and arranged her funeral down to the details about the music and pallbearers. Her husband concluded that she felt no hope for survival despite his encouragement to focus on life, not death. To his surprise and relief, as soon as the tasks were completed to her satisfaction, her mood lifted and she has felt optimistic ever since. Taking care of the "what if" freed her of this worry, leaving her more energy for hope. Even if her tumor had progressed despite treatment, getting her affairs in order would have made what time she had left less stressful. Had she died, her illness might have cut short the length of her life but not her expression of its closure.

In circumstances such as the example above, it's easy to see how preparing for the worst can free you to have hope. Many people understand the idea but simply can't do it by themselves; they need the support of others to make preparations. This reminds me of people who suffer needlessly from a toothache because they are afraid to go the dentist. When forced to go by a friend or relative, they obtain relief, feel grateful, and wish they'd gone sooner. If you want to prepare for the possibility of death but can't face it, get support from friends, family, or professionals.

This idea of preparing for the worst doesn't only apply to life-and-death concerns. Relatively minor challenges, too, may benefit from a "prepare for the worst and hope for the best" approach. For instance, if you are scheduled for a minor procedure to be done in day surgery, preparing for the possibility of needing an overnight stay at the hospital may relieve your anxiety about the care of your pet. If the consequences of unexpected problems are manageable when dealt with as they arise, then *not* preparing may be the best approach for you. If, however, the consequences of being unprepared for a poor outcome create a real crisis, this is not an approach that fosters Healthy Survivorship.

How do you feel about preparing for the worst? What are the consequences of not preparing? How hopeful are you about each of your goals? How optimistic are you about each of these goals?

Shifting Hopes

Hope is ever-changing, depending on many factors, some of which are beyond your control. In the early part of this chapter, factors that affect hopefulness were outlined, and ways to overcome obstacles to hopefulness were suggested. Getting good medical care can involve choosing to shift your level of hope over time. In going through my long series of recurrences and recoveries, I had times when I put some of my hopes on hold for a while. For instance, as I weighed my treatment options with my doctors, I let go of my hope to receive less toxic treatment when statistics suggested that more-toxic therapies would give me my best chance. When trying to stack the odds in my favor, I needed to base my treatment decision on dispassionate facts and not emotions like hope. Although a frightening and downright depressing process, I knew that making the most logical decision would give me the best chance—the most hope—of a good outcome. I also knew that the moment I made my decision, I could shift my emotional sense of hope into high gear. In 1991, when my treatments were working well but times were tough, hope guided me through and kept me from changing course or giving up prematurely. In 1995, when the first few cycles of chemotherapy weren't working well, my oncologist and I didn't let hopefulness keep us from recognizing the need to change my treatment plan.

You can choose to shift not only your level of hopefulness but also what you hope for. When I was first treated, I hoped for cure. When I was experiencing repeated recurrences, I hoped for relatively nontoxic therapies and longer remissions. When going through treatments, I hoped for a smooth course and a good response, and didn't worry too much about the long term. When in a remission, I hope for recovery from treatment and for the remission to last; I don't worry about whether I am cured. When I develop medical complications, I focus my hope on resolving the problems and getting back on course; my hopes for remission slip into the background for the time being. When I'm doing well medically and while I'm doing the things I need to do to get well, I choose to let my health-related hopes rest in the bottom of my hope chest. The main hopes that shape these days are ones that encourage me to live my life, such as my hope to embrace everyday opportunities to teach my children values and skills, to enjoy the company of a friend, learn something new, write another page of a book, play my violin, make a healthful and tasty dinner for my family, support a friend undergoing treatment, or take care of our garden. I hope to live life.

A common pitfall for survivors is hoping for the wrong things. On the one hand, hoping that your MRI scan was read wrong by the first doctor when you take it to a second doctor is a natural and adaptive hope. It helps you get through the shock while you are doing the right things to verify the diagnosis and move on. On the other hand, scheduling a consultation with your eighth specialist and pinning your hopes on the possibility that the first seven doctors who read your MRI are all wrong is to nourish a hope that will keep you from moving forward. Shifting your hopes to those like finding the most effective treatments, having treatments go smoothly, and seeing your condition respond well are hopes that help you.

So, how do you know what to hope for? Maybe you would find it helpful to create a Hope Tool for yourself. Outline in general terms what you would hope for in various situations. For example, you might ask yourself, "If I am going to die of this disease, what can I still hope for? If I am going to survive but have to deal with this as a chronic disease, what can I still hope for? If I am going to have a difficult treatment, what can I still hope for?" You can tailor the Hope Tool to your particular situation, concerns, and desires. For instance, if limb amputation is not needed now but is a possibility down the line, you might ask, "If I need amputation, what can I hope for?" Similarly, concerns close to your heart might cause you to ask, "What can I hope for if I can no longer have children? If I lose my voice? If I can no longer run a marathon or play the piano? If I lose my job or insurance?" Talking with other survivors and with friends and family may help you create a Hope Tool. A Hope

Hope is a choice. Choose hope.

Tool can help you open the door to hope in otherwise overwhelming situations. Knowing that you can find hope in almost any situation helps tame today's fears and nourishes Healthy Hope—the belief that you can do something to help your situation. Hope helps you get good care and live fully when you act on your hope in positive ways. The next chapter will talk about using your knowledge and hope to help you act effectively.

What does your Hope Tool look like?

Taking Action

I *knew exactly what I had to do to increase my chances of a good out-*
come. Without a doubt, doing the right things might help me. I
wanted to do all the right things. And yet, for some reason I was not
always doing the right things.

When you are sick, *what* you do affects *how well* you do. Although
obtaining sound knowledge and nourishing realistic hope are important
in and of themselves, the main way they help you is by enabling you to
take action that supports getting good care and living as fully as possible.
Effective action usually *follows* from knowledge and hope, but sometimes
you have to act simultaneously with, or even before you obtain knowledge or find hope. In the flurry of a new diagnosis or the crisis of a serious medical complication, you may know very little and understand even
less, but your condition may demand that you begin treatment immediately based on the expert advice of others. It may be only *after* you receive
your first few treatments that you begin to understand what happened
and what you can do to help your therapy work well. Or, what you may
need more than anything else to glimpse the first inklings of hope is to
get through your first few treatments. In general, however, and certainly
over the long run, knowledge and hope are the basis for action.

The problem is that having sound knowledge and solid hope doesn't automatically prompt, let alone guarantee, that you will take proper action. A wide variety of factors can keep you from acting on your knowledge and hope in healthy ways.

For starters, it can be hard work to do the right thing! *It is tough*—physically and emotionally—to prepare healthful meals and eat them when you are nauseated or to go through physical rehabilitation when you are weak. Meeting with a counselor can be trying. Working through emotional problems brought on by my illness was some of the hardest work I've ever done. To do the right thing can be uncomfortable, if not seemingly unbearable.

Before your diagnosis, you followed through on challenging ventures or dreadfully tedious tasks. You might expect that now you'd be very willing and able to make the sacrifices necessary to get well. But survivorship is complicated, and the path to recovery is strewn with barriers. Some obstacles to effective action are totally out of your control, such as if you have an allergy to the best drug for your condition. Others are very much in your control, such as getting beyond the fear of reporting a new symptom to your doctor. By this point you already possess basic knowledge and hope as described in earlier chapters. Now you need to know how to recognize obstacles to acting effectively, so that you can narrow the gap between knowing the right things to do and actually doing them.

Your "Final Answer"

"Is that your final answer?" is Regis Philbin's famous question on *Who Wants to Be a Millionaire*. It doesn't matter if the guest is confident of the answer or taking a wild guess. Nor does it matter if the contestant arrives at the answer alone, gets help from the audience, or takes two seconds versus two minutes to close in on an answer. The one and only factor that determines how much money the contestant takes home is his or her "final answer."

As a patient, *your actions* are your final answer. Your actions are the key force that shapes your physical reality. For instance, if you are experiencing the early signs of an allergic reaction, or some other problem for which your doctor has effective therapies, your knowledge of good treatment options doesn't help you if you stay home and do nothing. If you notify your doctor right away and then take your medications as prescribed, your knowledge can help you get well. Regarding nutrition, your liver cells don't know or care if your dentures don't fit anymore, or if you are losing thousands of calories every day to fever and diarrhea, or if you just feel too darned tired to eat.

> Your actions are your "final answer."

If you don't ingest enough food, your liver cells can't and won't make healing proteins; if you take in good-quality calories, your liver cells will help you heal. All that matters to your liver cells is what nutrients are delivered to them in your blood.

Action determines outcome on the nonmedical side, too. If tensions are mounting at home, your bounty of knowledge about healthy ways to communicate won't help at all if what you actually say and do incites hard feelings and makes your situation worse. Healthy responses build healthy relationships in hard times.

How often do your actions reflect what you know to be the best course?

The Gap between Knowledge and Action

Knowing what to do and doing it are two different things. I've watched respiratory therapists work up a sweat tending to patients who are on breathing machines for smoking-related emphysema, and then they gather outside the hospital during their break to light up cigarettes. I've read and heard accounts of experienced internists who are expert at recognizing the warning signs of heart attack and yet, after developing worrisome chest pain, pop antacid tablets all day, in one case even after a self-administered EKG heart tracing showed the classic changes of a heart attack!

Clearly, these experts have enough knowledge to be able to do the right things to protect their health. And, of course, this gap between knowledge and action is not peculiar to physicians. What's going on here? If people facing illness really want to get better and stay healthy, how can we explain the gap between knowing the best course of action and actually following it? My illness has provided many occasions for me to experience some of the common obstacles to acting effectively. As just one example, during a period of susceptibility to infection due to a profoundly low white count, I developed a painful swelling in my forearm and a low-grade fever. Unfortunately, it was near midnight. Aware of my increased risk of infection, I picked up the telephone receiver and dialed the first four digits of my doctor's telephone number. Then I hung up. My hand rested on the receiver where it stayed glued for who knows how long. Why? I didn't want to wake my doctor, but I also didn't want to take unnecessary risks or miss an opportunity to fix my arm easily. I felt torn between embarrassing myself by bothering my doctor with something he felt could have waited and waiting with something he would have wanted to see immediately. Nor could I bear the idea of worrying or upsetting my husband, calling a friend at midnight to watch my children, or bringing yet another complication to my doctor lest he get tired of taking care of my problems. Underlying everything was my primal fear: I didn't want to go back to the hospital. I didn't want to be sick again. So, after ten years of teaching other people how to be effective patients, I found it difficult to do the right thing. With ambivalence, I called.

Over the next few months of chemotherapy treatments, similar situations arose again and again. My decision-making delay was shortened with each successive problem. My anxiety lessened, too, but didn't go away. What helped me most was learning about my personal obstacles to acting effectively on my knowledge and hope, and finding ways to overcome them.

How large a gap is there between the measures you know will improve your health and what you do? What steps are you taking to improve your diet and sleep? Your exercise? What are some of the obstacles to effective action that you are facing?

Delays

Any problem that delays evaluating your condition, making a definitive diagnosis, mapping out a treatment plan, or getting you started on treatment can keep you from acting effectively. Some delays are inevitable and totally not your fault. These are not a problem in most cases. It's customary for patients to have to wait a few days for tests or their results, or to schedule an appointment in a week or two with a specialist for a second opinion. If anything, the short delay gives you time to begin adjusting to the changes while learning the basics about your situation and gathering your support group together. In contrast, when every single step of your evaluation takes a few weeks because of red tape, you need to push to get your tests scheduled sooner and results reported faster so that you can make some decisions and get started on treatment, if indicated. Don't hesitate to ask your primary-care physician or specialist to advocate on your behalf to help move the process along.

Whatever the problem, effective action depends on a team effort to make a correct diagnosis and determine the optimal treatment plan in a timely fashion. Since you are part of that team, you can become part of the difficulty. For instance, if you don't explain that you are having pain or trouble sleeping, nothing will be done to try to fix it. Or, if you report a problem but neglect to mention important pieces of information, your doctors may miss the diagnosis and consequently order more tests or decide to wait and see what happens instead of prescribing therapy. If your doctor reviews for you all your treatment options but you keep your questions and concerns to yourself, you may delay taking the next step because you feel unprepared to make a final decision or to schedule your first treatment. This might be a good time to review the information presented in chapter 3 on preventing and overcoming communication problems (page 86).

Tips for Minimizing Delays

- Explain as well as you can what problems you are having and what changes you are noticing (providing as many clues as possible).
- Make clear your needs and concerns regarding your evaluations and treatments.
- Work as a team player with your doctors and nurses to solve problems that arise and to prevent new problems.
- Ask your health-care team for help, if needed, to ensure timely tests, consultations, or treatments.

What steps can you take to minimize delays in making a diagnosis? Deciding on a course of treatment? Getting started on treatment?

Working the System

It is important to distinguish when *people* are making it hard for you versus when the problem lies with *the system* in which good people are working. Imagine a medical clinic where one nurse seems annoyed whenever you ask a question and never has time to answer adequately. If all the other nurses are happy to answer your questions to your satisfaction, the problem probably lies with that particular nurse. If, however, all the nice nurses in the office seem rushed and unable to take time to answer your questions, the problem is likely the system. Certainly, if you have to fill out a dozen forms and then wait forty-five minutes in a cold corridor for every blood test or scan, the problem lies with the system. In many cases, it is *your reaction* to a problem with the system that becomes the real obstacle to effective action. When you are sick, it doesn't help for you to get angry with the nurses for being overworked, your doctor for ordering the uncomfortable test, the receptionist for handing you the clipboard with the forms, or the technician for leaving you freezing in the hallway. What helps most is finding a response that best helps you now.

To illustrate this point further, imagine that your doctor's office routine includes having patients get undressed as soon as they are put in exam rooms. Let's say you resent or feel embarrassed wearing a flimsy examination gown when meeting and talking with your fully dressed doctors. What are you going to do about it? First, ask yourself, "Is the problem keeping me from getting good care?" If it's not, then decide how important the inequality is to you. If it's really not that big a deal, let it go. If it distresses you and you feel you'd be able to relate to your doctors better if you were wearing your street clothes, you can express your needs and assess their response. Your doctors and their staff may be accommodating, and your problem is over. If your doctors indicate difficulty with your request—perhaps it slows down the appointment—or they refuse to do it the way you prefer, for whatever reason, your response to the situation now can help or hurt you. If you choose to chalk up the tension regarding attire to a difference of opinion, you can get in the hospital gown and take advantage of the main reasons you like your physician— his or her fund of knowledge, skills, connections with institutions and specialists, experience treating people with your disease, and coverage by your insurance company. If, instead, you choose to dismiss your physician (a good doctor who could best help you), you become like drivers who enter an intersection because they have the right-of-way even though a speeding car is careening toward the same intersection: You get your way, but you jeopardize your well-being.

Weaknesses in the medical system upset patients. If you are unhappy or uncomfortable about some aspect of your care, ask yourself if you can find a better way to work within the system. Can you change how you do some things, or even just change your outlook in ways that help you? I never go for a medical appointment without a good book, and others are there listening to their Walkman or iPod. I see appointments as good reading time. Especially if you are compromised by illness, *you may be better off accepting and adjusting to an imperfect system that can help you in the long run* than trying to fix the day-to-day problems built into a system that is unjust or disrespectful but also can best help you get well.

> Everything does not have to run smoothly or be to your liking to turn out well.

As a physician, the problems with our conventional medical system pain me. They need to be fixed! Over time, I expect medical care in this country to become more patient focused in response to the effect of patients' demands on market forces. The issue for individual patients is timing and priorities. If a problem is not preventing you from obtaining treatment that can help you, what course of action will help you most, right now: working with the system or fighting it?

The equation tips in favor of your doing something if the problem with the system is keeping you from getting essential care. If your telephone calls aren't being returned or if your tests are not being ordered or done properly, it's time to speak with your doctor, write a letter, or do something else to make the system work better for you. In most cases, fixable problems will continue if you don't say or do anything. Many patients miss opportunities to take effective action because they are afraid that their complaints might offend their doctors or nurses, or jeopardize their care. Respectable doctors and nurses want and need to know about legitimate problems so they can work with you to fix them. You have a right to competent, timely, respectful care. (See The Patient's Bill of Rights, appendix V.)

Whenever you are telling a member of your health-care team about a problem, try to do it in a way that nourishes your alliance with them. Being a proverbial "thorn in the side" may cause your health-care team members to avoid you or want to dismiss you as a patient. Better to be a "squeaky wheel" that encourages your health-care team to better understand and respond to your legitimate requests and provide needed attention. Take a moment to distinguish whether a problem with the system is a temporary nuisance or injustice versus an important obstacle to your effective action. Then, choose the response that will best help you now.

What are your options when certain people *are keeping you from acting effectively? What are your options when* the system *is keeping you from acting effectively? When you have a problem with the system, are you a thorn in the side of your health-care team or are you a squeaky wheel that gets the grease?*

Too Tired

All action requires energy. If you are exhausted, how can you possibly do the things you know you need to do to get better and feel better? Suppose you're too tired to eat the type and amount of food that could improve your energy. With fewer good-quality calories onboard, you feel even more tired, which causes you to eat even less, progressing into a vicious cycle. Or you feel too wiped out to move, so you don't get any exercise, leading to progressive deconditioning that makes you feel even more tired. Since fatigue is such a common symptom in patients during and after illness, minimizing physical fatigue is often an essential element to acting effectively.

> Illness-related fatigue is different from the tiredness that healthy people feel.

Tips for Dealing with Illness-Related Fatigue
- Remind yourself that illness-related fatigue and treatment-related fatigue are real and different from the tiredness that healthy people feel at the end of a long day.
- Learn about things you can do to lessen fatigue; work with your doctors and nurses to improve your energy level.
- Recognize how your fatigue is impeding effective action.
- Start slowly and build up; take the first small step *today.*
- Enlist friends and family to help you get started and stay motivated.

What healing measures are being impeded by your fatigue?

The Mighty Dollar

Money, or lack of it, can be a formidable foe of effective action. Health care is expensive. Your budget might have been tightly strapped before your illness. Even when you have excellent insurance, out-of-pocket medical and nonmedical expenses such as travel costs and child care can create obstacles to taking advantage of available treatments and services. You have a right to effective treatment. Many people and organizations are working hard to protect your rights. When money is an obstacle, contact people who can help you understand and pursue options for gaining access to effective treatments. To begin, ask the staff in your physician's office to explain your payment options and refer you to people who can offer advice and support. Via phone or e-mail, contact the local and national survivor organizations as discussed in chapter 3.

Money issues can create emotional barriers to effective action even when you have easy access to top-of-the-line medical care. If people have trouble talking about money matters under normal circumstances, the setting of illness can make this topic even harder to discuss. How dare you or a family member grumble about the financial burden of medical treatments that might make your life longer or more comfortable? What do you say when your spouse, after months and months of caring for your children and supporting your every need, suddenly and without consulting with you goes out and buys a boat to celebrate the end of your treatments?

What about the money concerns that arise after you've experienced a medical false alarm? Although everyone is telling you that you did the right thing when you called your doctor complaining of abdominal pain that turned out to be gas, resentment and guilt may intensify when expensive bills for that emergency-room visit start trickling in. It's obvious why you might hesitate to let anyone know the next time you develop a new symptom. You *know* you should call the doctor, but you are worried that you'll end up wasting more money if it turns out to be another false alarm or—worse!—it turns out to be a real problem that will bring with it additional medical bills for a long time, if not forever after. Hence, your anxieties about money steer you to keep your symptoms secret. You justify it to yourself with the perilous decision "I'll wait a while and see if it goes away."

Money also can keep you from taking advantage of healing measures intended to help you feel better and support your medical treatments. In an attempt to minimize expenses, you might skimp on food, comfort aids, or medications prescribed to control pain or other side effects. To do so would be like buying a nice car but not buying enough gas to get where you want to go. The measures prescribed and recommended to support your well-being are important parts of your overall treatment plan. The cost of supportive therapies and tending to your nonmedical needs are part of your overall cost of treatment.

As for managing all the nonmedical stresses that arise when dealing with family illness, money can be a third rail. A casual mention of a cash matter can trigger arguments about family members' roles, responsibilities, actions, and attitudes. If your family's money issues are complicated or emotional, talk with your doctor and nurse about a referral to professionals who can help you understand and talk about these charged topics. Not only may this help free you from unnecessary financial burdens; it will also encourage you to gain additional insight into how the illness is affecting you and your family. Understanding and support can lead you to find healthy ways to cope and grow.

What money issues are obstacles to your taking effective action?

Two Steps Forward, One Step Back

Setbacks and failures can slow or stop your progress. From a purely practical point of view, it takes time to learn what you need to know when events necessitate a change in game plan. In many cases, however, the real obstacle is not so much the effort required to make the shift but your reaction to the setback or failure. Let's say you suffer an unusual side effect from a medicine and your doctor prescribes a different one. If you don't begin the new medicine because you're afraid of developing untoward side effects, your emotional reaction to the problem with the first medicine has become an obstacle to effective action now. Setbacks and failures are common features in the landscape of survivorship, occurring even when everyone does everything perfectly right. Don't let problems keep you from moving forward. For example, if your partner gets testy for a while after you attempt to talk through some differences of opinion, your relationship still can end up in a better place in the long run. Keep trying.

What if setbacks and rough spots are your fault? You may try to increase your exercise too quickly and end up pulling a muscle or overtiring yourself. You could take a nutritional supplement that interferes with your treatment or precipitates a complication. If you screw up, what now? As discussed in chapter 7, beating up on yourself is a mistake. Forgive yourself, learn from the mistake, and move forward.

With so many things changing and going on during your evaluation, treatment, and recovery, it's inevitable that some things won't go smoothly. You're going to make some mistakes and hit some bumps in the road. Setbacks and failed attempts can become serious obstacles to effective action if you don't learn from them and you keep making the same mistakes over and over. A failed attempt doesn't mean that *you* are a failure. It means the attempt failed. *You* don't fail until you stop trying. As a Healthy Survivor, keep setbacks and failures from becoming obstacles to effective action.

How do you feel when your attempt to get better, or to make things better in some way, fails? How does it make you feel about trying a new approach?

Full Moons and Black Cats

Plain old bad luck can be an obstacle to effective action. If you get sick at night and your local twenty-four-hour pharmacy is out of stock of a particular drug, you may have to suffer until morning when a store opens that carries your medication. If your car develops a flat tire on the way to your doctor's appointment, you may have to reschedule for another day. On the nonmedical front, if the family counselor you'd most like to see is out of town for a few weeks, you have to either delay your first session or consult with someone else.

Bad luck is not your fault! And when something goes awry it's not because there's a full moon or because you crossed paths with a black cat. Bad luck is a part of life. Everyone has bad luck at times. If you feel that you're having more than the usual amount of rotten luck while going through serious illness, this may be because you have fewer reserves to deal with ordinarily occurring problems. Or it may be because you feel particularly vulnerable and insecure. Or it may be that, indeed, you are having an unusually long and deep streak of bad luck.

Handles for Times When Nothing Seems to Go Right

- Unexpected life challenges are just that: *challenges* to be faced and overcome, and not "punishment" for past wrongdoing or arbitrary "tests" of character.
- Life is a game of shifting priorities; right now, I need to get through the most pressing problems.
- Having a bit of bad luck doesn't mean I am unlucky; it means that I live in a world where unlucky things happen.
- Bad luck can be followed by good luck.

Do you feel lucky or unlucky? How is this changing how you are dealing with your illness?

Strategically Using Your Emotions

Bad luck, money problems, setbacks, and failures are examples of external problems that, when mired in your emotions, can become serious obstacles to effective action. Emotions play such a dominant role in widening the gap between knowledge and action that the next few sections will look at a few of them more closely. As a Healthy Survivor, it matters less what emotions you experience than how your emotions affect what you do. As a Healthy Survivor, channel your emotions in ways that help you act.

This brings me to a paradox of Healthy Survivorship: Doing a good job of channeling your emotions in healthy ways invariably includes times of forgiving yourself for doing a bad job of channeling your emotions. You're human. Nobody does exactly the right thing at exactly the right time in every situation, and certainly not when health is involved. Emotions have a way of confusing the picture and keeping you from responding to situations the way you want to or know is best. For me, I suspect perfection in action would only be achieved at the expense of my spontaneity, creativity, and passion. I could fill an entire book with stories of times I've known what to do and yet didn't do it. As a patient, my goal has been to narrow the gap: to maximize the times my emotions are helping me and to minimize the times they are hurting me, especially when the stakes are high.

Who's in Control?

Serious illness is notorious for making patients feel that they've lost control over their world. From the mundane task of going to the grocery store to the monumental mission of planning your future, your normal sense of order and predictability is disrupted by a diagnosis of serious illness. Medical evaluations and treatments put extra demands on your time and energy and load you with more worries. Your health-care team is calling most of the shots, telling you to do specific things at specific times at specific places in specific ways. And, no matter how confident you feel about what you are doing, you can't control how your body will respond. This inability to predict if your upcoming course will be smooth or if things will turn out well can make you feel out of control.

What is your response to feeling out of control? If you become overwhelmed, you may be like the patient who got stuck, unable to decide on a course of treatment. Other patients who feel overwhelmed stop eating or don't take their medications properly. If hopelessness and loss of confidence are your reactions to feeling out of control, you may become like the patients who give up and don't make any effort to find out about treatment options. You may make no effort to adjust to the many unwanted changes. If the loss of control makes you angry, you may lash out at those people who can help you most.

Some patients try to regain a sense of control at any cost. One nineteen-year-old patient with leukemia regularly hops on his motorcycle despite emphatic warnings that his low platelet count puts him at grave risk of bleeding from even minor trauma. Another patient continues to smoke, maintaining a sense of command over *something* in a situation that feels out of control. Yet another patient pursues an expensive bogus antiarthritis cream because he is comforted by his sense of taking charge of his recovery. The problem, of course, is that these patients *feel* in control when in actuality their actions give them *less* control over their outcome than if they'd pursued measures that, although not guaranteed, were proven safe and effective.

Problems arise when the best course of action is to "hurry up and do nothing." Patients who need to feel in control often want to *do something*, not sit back and wait. The power of this desire has been supported by a research study looking at patients who were taking a nutritional supplement in hopes of alleviating symptoms of a chronic condition. After being shown solid scientific data that the supplement was harmless but had no beneficial effect for their condition, the patients continued to take the expensive supplement. Why? The results of this fascinating study suggest that when people feel vulnerable or are in pain, their emotional need to *do something* usurps their rationality. Taking such therapies is not a big problem if your physicians say they are safe and you are taking them in addition to the best proven therapies (and as long as you don't have to mortgage your house to pay for them). It's another story if you are pursuing a worthless therapy *instead of* effective therapy, or if you are pursuing any unproven therapy that can cause harm. In these cases, your desire to feel in control—to feel proactive—is sabotaging actions that could help you. As a Healthy Survivor, make sure that actions that enhance your sense of feeling in control are, in fact, giving you some control.

When does the desire to feel confident and in control lure you toward measures that might hurt you? How can you adjust to lack of control? How can you satisfy your need to feel in control?

Control is not all-or-nothing. As a physician—as a person!—I'd long understood and believed that individuals can't have *total* control over their medical outcome, whatever they believe. My years as a doctor had convinced me that luck, genetics, the environment, and a host of unexplained factors interplay at the controls of our lives. Yet, for a short while after my second recurrence, I found myself tempted by the self-help literature on alternative methods for curing cancer. They offered me something I wanted and wasn't quite ready to give up—a sense of complete control over my disease and its outcome. My sudden interest in unscientific methods of healing left me feeling confused, disheartened, and insecure about my role in my healing. Just knowing in my head that I couldn't have total control didn't bring me peace. As a patient, I also had to accept in my heart that total control is impossible before I could be released from the grip of false hope and set free to experience the rich hope of effective action. Paradoxically, when I let go of the comforting illusion of total control I felt *more* in control than ever, and I was able to maximize my control.

In 1995, Jane Brody in her *New York Times* column printed my answer to the question of whether I thought my remission would last: "We'll find out as I not 'wait and see' but 'live and see.'" Soon thereafter, I received an irate letter from a patient with a brain tumor chastising me for not encouraging survivors to be absolutely confident about a good outcome. It wasn't the first time a patient had reproached me for setting my sights too low. But it takes a lot of emotional, physical, and spiritual energy to deny something you know to be true. In 1995, my frequent recurrences and decreasing treatment options put me in a statistical group of patients with a poor long-term outcome. For me to maintain total confidence that I was cured of my disease would have demanded that I contradict what I knew: that I was human and vulnerable, that most other people in my situation do not live long lives, and that it *was possible* for me to die of my disease. Instead of living with the psychological tension inherent in denying the possibility, I let go of my desire to feel completely in control. The result? Far from feeling hopeless, I felt relieved and energized! All my energy that would have been wasted trying to convince myself of something that I knew wasn't true could now be directed toward healing measures such as a healthy diet, good-quality sleep, regular exercise, a sense of peacefulness, and, importantly, nourishing hope of a complete recovery.

> Letting go of the illusion of *complete* control puts you in a position to *increase* control over your situation.

How much control do you believe you can have over the ultimate outcome? How much control do you feel you need?

Controlling Control

Letting go of control can be an effective way to gain control. Undergoing general anesthesia is not an everyday event but illustrates the point: You have to be willing to let others control your breathing—your very life—before you can enjoy the benefits of major surgery. In a less dramatic way, your medical exams, procedures, and office visits tend to go more smoothly when you willingly submit to others' schedules, requests, pokings and proddings, styles of communication, invasions of privacy, and sometimes unpleasant demands. As long as your health-care team's requests are reasonable and respectful, by doing what you can to increase their ability to help you, letting go of control helps you.

When I worked as a doctor, one of the night nurses nicknamed me "Dr. Vampire" because I was slick with a needle and could draw blood from patients who had tiny, scarred veins. So, naturally, it was hard for me as a patient to sit back and watch someone else stick my arm. If I tried to control the situation by directing the technician and scrutinizing his or her every move, I made things worse. In this situation, it was usually better for everyone when I just shut up and maybe even turned my head to signal my letting go. Left alone to do their work, the phlebotomists did a better job. Letting go of control helped me.

Knowing how much to let go and when to let go take judgment. Beware of letting go *too much* or *too early*. I mentioned earlier how I keep quiet when I have my blood drawn. Let me explain further so that you don't get the mistaken impression that I leave myself unnecessarily vulnerable. First, it helps to understand that the routine of drawing blood has been a big deal for me because I am what nurses call "a hard stick." Many of the veins in my hands and arms, which were small before my diagnosis, became scarred by months of caustic chemotherapy. Consequently, when I go for blood tests, *before* I shut up and turn my head I take some control by mentioning to the phlebotomist which of my veins usually works the best. If the phlebotomist

> Letting go at the right time can help you regain some control.

chooses to ignore my advice, I may think that he or she is making a mistake, but I let it go, anyway. Most times, the technicians successfully draw blood from their chosen vein. If, however, the needle is still hurting after the initial stab (it shouldn't hurt), or if the phlebotomist is taking too long, or I see that the needle is going in too deep or at a bad angle, I politely yet firmly take back control by asking him or her to please stop and get someone else to draw my blood. So, you see, as I go through the blood-drawing process, I experience a constant fluctuation of control.

In any situation that requires action, the key question is this: What will help me most at this moment in this particular instance? If letting go is best, being passive is the best way to act effectively. If letting go increases my risk of problems, being too passive becomes an obstacle to getting optimal care, and I have to be proactive. Healthy Survivors modulate the ebb and flow of control in ways that maximize their chance of a good outcome in each situation.

In what situations do you let go too much? In what situations do you let go too early? How do you decide when it is right for you to let go?

The Only Thing We Have to Fear

Franklin Roosevelt's words during the heart of the Great Depression speak well to people facing serious illness: "The only thing we have to fear is fear itself." Fear can be one of the biggest obstacles to effective action, especially since it can be silent, insidious, and can masquerade as anger or another emotion. As discussed in chapter 7, fear is the normal, healthy response to perceived danger. Unfortunately, fear can keep you from acting in ways that might help your situation.

Early in my illness, fear was making it difficult for me to sleep, eat, or enjoy anything. My mistake was thinking that I had to get rid of my fears before I could act effectively. It takes time to tame fear. In 1993, I didn't have that time; I had to decide soon on a course of treatment and proceed. The advice given by the Wizard to the Cowardly Lion in Baum's *The Wizard of Oz* provided me with just the inspiration I needed to make a decision and face more treatment: "True courage is in facing danger when you are afraid." With great relief, I realized that I didn't have to eliminate my fear to move forward. My shaky signature on the informed-consent form enabled me to enjoy the benefits of the clinical trial just as much as if my penmanship had been sure and steady.

True courage is taking proper action when you feel afraid.

You can take action when you are afraid. But it's awfully draining to keep this up for weeks or months at a time. As a Healthy Survivor, taming fear is an important task. For me, the first steps toward taming my fears include letting my fears surface in safe places (at home with my husband and close friends; in the hospital with my doctors, nurses, and oncology social workers; in my journal; in my private prayers), acknowledging my fears to myself, and sharing my fears with someone who cares.

Another approach that often works well for me is to act braver than I feel and, as advised in *The King and I,* whistle a happy tune. Trying to *appear* unafraid when frightened out of my wits seems to initiate a positive feedback loop: I feel a bit braver, which makes it easier to act confident, which helps me feel more confident, which helps me take action that requires courage.

Tips for Overcoming Fear That Is Blocking Effective Action

- *Stay focused on your main health goal: getting better.* More than wanting to avoid doctor visits, diagnostic tests, surgeries, missing special events, and so on, you want to do the right things to get better.
- *Talk with other survivors who've experienced the same fears.* Seeing someone on the other side of treatment, or even just hearing someone else's success story, can help tame fear by reinforcing the belief in the possibility of a good outcome. It can nourish your hope of getting through, too.
- *Ask a friend or family member to accompany you to tests, office visits, or treatments, or arrange to meet for lunch or a movie afterward.* The company of friends and family helps tame fears by distracting, comforting, encouraging, and just being with you.
- *Think about how your loved ones would feel if you didn't do the right things to get well.* Or think about how *you'd* feel if your loved ones allowed fear to keep them from getting needed medical attention.
- *Think about the difference in likely outcomes depending on if you do the right thing or don't do it.* The idea of preventable problems getting out of hand is scarier than facing short-term challenges.
- *Reframe the issue as a test situation: Question #1, "What is the right thing to do?" Question #2, "Am I doing the right thing?"* This approach reduces an emotional hodgepodge of feelings to a logical test with right and wrong answers. Your desire to get the answer right and do the right thing can help to overcome fear.

*What steps can you take to tame fears that are keeping you
from acting effectively?*

Anger

Anger, like fear, is a normal emotion with a bad reputation in social
circles. Just as you are urged to "Be brave!" and "Be positive!" you are
encouraged to control or hide any anger. Certainly, in the context of
acting effectively when you are sick, anger can create serious problems.
Recognizing and understanding your anger, and knowing how to manage
and channel it, will help prevent anger from becoming an obstacle to
effective action. Anger can hurt your ability to get good care when it

- causes the members of your health-care team to withdraw their attention and, possibly, services;
- makes it difficult for friends and family to understand you or be supportive;
- clouds your decision making;
- makes you feel sick or get sick;
- makes it hard for you to eat well or sleep well;
- keeps you from complying with effective therapies;
- makes you feel hopeless or helpless.

If you find yourself steamed about something that you *could* fix but at
too great a cost, find a way to calm your anger and channel the energy into
something that helps you now. Maybe joining an art group will channel
your energy into creativity. In a pottery class, you can release anger by hit-
ting and molding the clay. Many patients find that "giving back" helps. One
danger of this approach is when your altruistic efforts and sense of purpose
divert your attention from everyday efforts that will help you get better.
Volunteering all day for service organizations, talking at all hours with
other survivors in need, and training for marathons to raise money for
research are all noble causes, but they impede your healing if they interfere

with your eating well or sleeping enough, relating to your family and friends, or getting needed respite from the seriousness of illness.

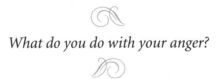

What do you do with your anger?

To Trust or Not to Trust

Trust paves the way to effective action. Trust—the belief that someone or something can be relied upon—begins with self-trust. If you have a "feeling" that the ache in your shoulder is important or the dose of your pill is not right, believe what you are seeing or feeling. Trust your intuition and act on it by calling your doctor. If it is a false alarm, that's okay. Don't let a false alarm erode your self-trust or keep you from acting effectively the next time you note a worrisome physical change.

In addition to trusting yourself, you have to trust the members of your health-care team. If you think, even for a moment, that your doctors or nurses will be annoyed at you for calling, you may hesitate to call about something that isn't clearly a life-threatening emergency. If you doubt the competence of any member of your health-care team, you may not follow their advice. If, for whatever reason, you can't trust your health-care team, you need to find a new team.

Trust is a two-way process. Effective action depends on your doctors and nurses being able to trust you to communicate honestly with them and comply with their advice or let them know why you can't or won't. Trust affects all aspects of healing, not just the physical side. When you don't trust a family member to respond in caring ways, you might keep to yourself some news or worries that you are better off sharing. Or you might decide to try to solve a problem or run an errand on your own that puts your health at risk.

One of the most poignant moments in my entire survivorship occurred a few months into my illness. My blood counts were low, and my three kids all had runny noses. I was off in our bedroom while Ted was bathing our two girls. William, a toddler, was in the next room where Ted could keep an eye on him. When William bumped his head and began wailing, Ted wisely finished rinsing off the girls so he could get them safely out of the tub before turning his attention to William. The problem was me: I heard my baby's screams and, against medical advice, I opened the bedroom door and headed toward the family room. Ted scooped up the two girls in his arms and intercepted me, screaming, "Wendy, get away!" Later that night, at a quieter moment, he bared his soul and told me that he could handle everything but my putting myself at risk.

This incident had a host of different emotions playing into it, but I tell it here to illustrate the central role of trust. I needed to trust Ted to take care of the kids and the house, even if he did things differently than I did and even if things didn't get done as quickly or as well. I also needed to trust that Ted understood and accepted that I couldn't carry my load of chores or child care as if I were well. Most important of all, Ted needed to trust me that I would do whatever I could do to help my physical recovery. From Ted's point of view, the worst thing I could do to him or our children was to unnecessarily jeopardize my health.

You may have to take a leap of faith and expect people who care to respond in helpful ways. With time, you'll discover who can deal with your illness and your varied needs, and who can't. Unlike your expert and experienced doctors and nurses who have a professional obligation to be trustworthy, some of your friends and family members may start to run from the whole situation. Many only need a bit of guidance and encouragement from you, and they'll be able to rise to the occasion. Other people just won't or can't; you'd be wasting your time and energy trying to reach them. Don't fall into the trap of automatically blaming yourself, thinking that you must be too self-centered or complaining too much. Don't hesitate to ask for needed support from people who can help.

> Trust is vital to Healthy Survivorship.

How well do you trust yourself? Your health-care team? Do you draw on your trust of family and friends to stand by your side?

Wishing on Stars

A dangerous obstacle to effective action is magical thinking, namely, believing in the ability to manipulate natural forces through symbols or rituals. This usually involves believing in "cause and effect" when, in fact, two events are totally unrelated. Magical thinking can help you or hurt you, depending on how it affects your actions. If knocking on wood tames your anxiety when someone mentions a potential problem, go ahead and rap your knuckles on some furniture. If your confidence is buoyed by the fact that you are receiving treatment on the clinic's eighteenth floor, and eighteen is your lucky number, that's fine, too. The problem arises when magical thinking leads you to knock on wood *instead of* calling your doctor with a new symptom or to choose a particular treatment *solely because* it is administered in a clinic housed on the eighteenth floor. Now magical thinking is hurting you by impeding effective action.

When faced with a potential problem, such as a new lump, some people enter a mode of magical thinking: "If I go to a doctor, then this lump might be serious." They don't mention the lump to anyone or do anything about it, comforted by the belief that if they act as if the lump is nothing important, it can't be serious (or maybe they don't even have a lump!). In most cases, this illogical magical thinking is completely subconscious and only lasts a few hours or days. But it can be powerful enough to cause a delay in evaluation, especially since fear is usually playing a role.

Wishful thinking can interfere with effective action in all areas of life. It can cause a patient, devastated by an unwanted divorce, to come alive with newfound hope that the diagnosis of life-threatening disease will prompt the "ex" to want to come back. Wishful thinking leads responsible parents to believe that their illness is not affecting their kids. These parents take no steps to help their children understand and cope with the changes. As with other potential obstacles to effective action, the central issue is recognizing when magical thinking is playing a role in your decisions and determining whether magical thinking is helping you or harming you.

When do you use magical thinking? Does it ever hamper effective action?

The Ostrich Syndrome

When people act as if all is well when, in fact, something is wrong, they are said to be exhibiting the "ostrich syndrome" because of the tale that an ostrich will bury its head in the sand when confronted with something unpleasant. The problem, of course, is that the unpleasant reality is still there, in many cases progressing unhampered. Running away from problems and denying problems can become serious obstacles to effective action. Chapter 8 discusses the difference between denial and repression, and how to use repression in healthy ways. You need to know if denial might be preventing effective action. Are your views clashing with the judgment and advice of those who care about you? Are family members pushing you to eat more or exercise more than you think you need to? Do you sense tension with close friends when you discuss your intention to return to work soon? Are your doctors suggesting you see a counselor or take medication for depression when you think you are fine? If you sense conflict but feel confident you know what's best for you, you might be absolutely right! But you might be dangerously wrong. Enlist the expertise of an impartial professional counselor who can help you arrive at the truth about what you need to do to get better.

What issues seem to cause tension between you and your family? In the past, have you been able to push worrisome or awful things out of your mind easily?

How Embarrassing!

"Mom! I can't be seen by my friends using one of those!" My teenage daughter rolled her eyes, exasperated with my lack of fashion sense. She then ran out the front door into the pouring rain, leaving behind her umbrella. An analogous scene is played out in many physicians' offices. The doctor asks, "How are you feeling?" and the patient who is suffering from troublesome symptoms responds, "Fine, just fine." A million reasons explain this common response, including wanting to avoid appearing to anyone, including yourself, as alarmist, ignorant, or whiny. The problem is that appearing "fine" can keep you from feeling well by keeping you from getting the care you need. Situations that can be particularly embarrassing and prompt you to withhold information from your health-care team or family include times when you are

- not complying completely with your treatment;
- adjusting your medications, diet, or activity level without supervision;
- using alternative therapy;
- feeling too anxious to wait for the next scheduled checkup;
- harboring doubts regarding your doctor's advice or conclusions;
- feeling pressure from your family or friends to question your doctor;
- feeling less brave or optimistic than everyone seems to expect you to be.

Since I'm a physician who knows when a symptom is wacky, I was exceedingly self-conscious when I developed a strange symptom during one of my courses of treatments. I dealt with my discomfort by prefacing my disclosure, "Doctor, I feel embarrassed about what I'm going to tell you," and then described the odd but real symptom. It helped us both deal with something uncomfortable.

Another time I dealt with my self-consciousness with humor. The researcher of the clinical trial in which I was treated in 1994 needed a lymph tissue sample from a node under my armpit. He found it easiest and safest if I sat up straight with my hand on the nape of my neck, and my elbow up and extended as far back as I could. So, while striking the position of a femme fatale, I told the doctor, "You know, Doctor, I don't pose like this for just anyone!" I was terribly self-conscious until I said to myself, "I'm a patient. This is a medical setting. I am helping my doctor get a specimen of cancer." Whether using humor or distracting conversation, I held still so he could get it over with as quickly as possible.

Tips for Taming Self-Consciousness in Medical Settings

- Your relationship with your physicians and nurses is professional, not social.
- You help your doctors find answers for you when you provide the most complete and accurate information.
- Maximizing your health often involves doing things you would never do in a social situation, and doing things that are against your nature.
- Success is measured by increasing your chances of a good outcome, not by improving your outer appearance.

A common situation where self-consciousness becomes an obstacle to effective action is when patients don't understand something about their condition or treatment but don't ask for clarification for fear of looking dumb. You have a right to understand what's happening to you. You need to understand what you are supposed to do. Don't ever guess at what was said or what you are supposed to do because you might guess wrong. Ask.

When talking about your health or undergoing tests and procedures, self-consciousness can hurt you if it affects what you say and how you act.

What steps can you take to keep embarrassment from becoming an obstacle to effective action?

Second Nature

Habits are behaviors that you do automatically. Good habits are practiced behaviors that help you act effectively by saving you time, effort, or energy needed to make a new decision each time you are in a similar situation. Habits are especially protective when your instincts and emotions might steer you otherwise. A classic example is learning to "Stop, drop, and roll!" if your clothing catches fire. You have to suppress your natural urge to run, which would only fan the flames and worsen the threat. *Knowing* what to do is a good start, but you have to *practice* the technique to make it familiar enough to do in an emergency.

An examination of your habits in the context of illness may reveal routines that are no longer serving you well. Some habits that helped me work as a physician became obstacles to effective action when I became a patient. For instance, drinking coffee in response to feeling sleepy was an appropriate and adaptive response when I was on call and had to drive to the emergency room to see a patient. Drinking coffee was not a healthy response to my afternoon tiredness when dealing with chemo; rather, I did best to listen to my body and take a nap. Or, when evaluating my patients, the ingrained reflex of methodically considering every possible medical complication or problem that could arise helped me do a good job. When going through my cancer treatments, I could make myself crazy thinking of potential problems all the time. I needed to develop new habits instead of analyzing every little sneeze.

Reassess your habits. What are your habits for eating? Sleeping? Preparing for doctor visits? Telling family about setbacks? It takes time and effort to break old habits and create new ones. Before your diagnosis, chances are you were not in the habit of writing down when you took an occasional over-the-counter medication. If you are now taking a number of medications, doing so is a good idea. So is going to bed earlier than before. Be patient with yourself, and practice, practice, practice. Every time you do the right thing, you make it a little easier to do the right thing the next time. The more deep-seated your new habit becomes, the more likely it will help when you are not thinking clearly, and when fear and instincts push you to act otherwise.

What old habits—for example, sleep habits—may not be in your best interest now? What new habits would help you act effectively?

Ruling Yourself

Rules are a set of laws you create to help you act effectively in situations where fatigue or your emotions might lead you to break a healthy habit and do something unwise. In situations where you don't have a habit, good rules eventually lead to good habits that help you get good care and live fully. Some rules are dictated by your health-care team, such as "Call the office if your temperature goes above 101 degrees." Other rules are designed at your discretion, helping you relate to your loved ones, take good care of yourself between doctor visits, and deal with the risks and uncertainty of recovery.

Rules have a bad reputation. When you were a child, most of the rules governing your life were set by adults, and not enjoyed. ("Finish your homework before you watch television.") Even when you appreciate that rules are intended to protect or help you in some way, they can feel restrictive, especially those that begin "Don't" or "You can't." For many

> Good rules are good friends.

people, children and adults alike, the notion of rules stirs immediate negative feelings.

In a risk-filled world, good rules are good friends. I have believed this wholeheartedly since the time I chose to break one of our cardinal family rules: "*Never* eat or drink near the computers." One afternoon, anticipating a family outing to the park and concerned about a deadline for an article, I broke the rule. Carrying my cupful of soup into my study, I reassured myself, "I'll be careful and won't spill it." And I didn't spill a single drop. Unfortunately, my daughter sprang into my study to show me a picture, and the corner of her book caught the handle of my mug, tipping it toward my computer. As if in slow motion, hot tomato soup doused the keyboard of my new laptop!

Ever since that electronic disaster, I've appreciated how good rules are good friends. Rules protect me, but only if I obey them. Far from being restrictive, rules set me free by saving me from wasting energy deciding what to do in a situation where there is only one smart choice. Rules help me resist the ever-present temptation to go against my better instincts. When I choose to follow them, rules save me from dealing with many avoidable problems.

Wendy's Rules for Dealing with Your Health-Care Team

- If you note something that *might* need immediate attention, notify your health-care team right away no matter what time of day or night it is.
- If you note something that doesn't appear to be an emergency, call your doctor during office hours.
- If you note something new but it doesn't appear to be significant, give yourself a reasonable target date, such as three days or a week. If, at the appointed date, the change persists, connect with your health-care team about it. If it gets worse before the target date, call right away.
- Whenever you are not sure if a symptom is important or not, call your doctors and let them decide.
- If you are experiencing an emotion that is making it harder to do the right thing, acknowledge your emotional discomfort. Make your emotional discomfort clear to your doctors and nurses, and family or friends who might be involved in the evaluation and treatment of this problem.
- Make pacts with your close friends: You will call them for help if you are having trouble doing what you know to be the right thing, and they will help you do the right thing. As a safeguard against imposing, your friends and family members should promise to tell you when they need you to lean on someone else at the moment.

For me, one huge advantage of having rules is that emotional medical issues are reduced to a simple objective question: Do I want to follow my rule? Since I trust my rules to protect me and since I've always been someone who liked getting the "right" answer, this technique helps me.

When dealing with illness, the benefit of good rules extends beyond medical situations. Before my diagnosis, my husband and I were comfortable with our ability to share concerns and problems. After cancer, the equation changed: Voicing any concern triggered a highly emotional reaction in my husband and set off a cascade of emotions in both of us. When I'd develop a new symptom, I no longer knew the best timing or way to tell Ted. In addition to the original problem causing me to worry, I worried about how and when to bring Ted into the picture. I needed a rule. So, Ted and I agreed that when either of us notices a change or a problem, or if we are worried about something, we share our concerns with the other sometime before going to sleep that night. No matter how silly or serious the concern, and no matter how good or bad a time to add another problem to our plate, we tell the other what is worrying us. This mutually agreed-upon rule saves us from surprise revelations about any problems that have been brewing for a while. Ever since, neither of us ever wonders or worries that a potential problem is being kept secret by the other.

My rules make life easier for me and help me do the right things for my health. I've found that as soon as I share news of a potential problem and decide on a course of action, most problems (even potentially serious ones) seem to demand less attention and cause less stress. My sense of isolation, fear, and lack of control is minimized. Good rules help me act on my knowledge and hope in effective ways.

What are your rules for responding to a new symptom or medical concern? For sharing concerns with loved ones?

Bending with the Wind

One thing you can depend on in life: Nothing stays the same. Implicit in my advice to develop healthy habits and create healthy rules is the notion of flexibility, an essential trait for Healthy Survivorship. An approach or style that works best in one situation may be counterproductive in another. Habits work best if you know when it's time to let go of current habits—even if they are still relatively new—and create new habits. Rules work best if you recognize the *rare* occasions when they need to be broken. Flexibility is a virtue. As a Healthy Survivor, flexibility is essential if you want to take advantage of the benefits of taking control *and* letting go, waiting patiently *and* approaching problems proactively, and acting independently *and* accepting support. Like the wings of birds in flight, flexibility can set you free.

Rambo

Doing the right thing matters more than how you get yourself to do the right thing. As discussed in chapter 7, accepting support when you need support is a sign of strength, not weakness.

Tips for Accepting Support

- Leaning on someone's arm may enable you to stand up and take your first steps toward regaining your muscle strength and balance.
- Accepting emotional support when you get bad news may pull you through your grief and confusion as smoothly as possible so you can move forward.
- Asking for companionship may combat your loneliness.
- Confiding in someone who cares and understands may tame your fears and reveal the courage needed to proceed with tests or treatments.

> The Rambo approach may get you through, but accepting help leads to a safer, easier, and less frightening journey.

- Sharing your goals with a confidante may engender a sense of accountability and inspire you to follow through to the end.
- Venting your complaints may release your anger and channel your energies toward recovery.
- Accepting help with household chores or child care may preserve your energy for life-enhancing tasks.
- Accepting medications for pain, anxiety, insomnia, depression, or poor appetite may renew the strength needed to make wise decisions and act on them.

How often do you lean on others? Whom do you lean on?

Reach for the Stars

Healthy goals can motivate you to take effective action. Sometimes, all you need to do to overcome obstacles to action is sit down and articulate your goals. Long-term goals such as getting well or returning to work establish a useful foundation that can be used as inspiration when you are tempted to act in self-defeating ways. Intermediate goals such as getting through your current round of treatment also help pull you into tomorrow. Realistic short-term goals—calling a friend, doing one load of laundry, eating well *today*, or creating a list of your long-term goals—serve an especially important role because they tend to be more concrete, and because you usually have more control over their outcome. The zing of success can energize you and nourish your hope, creating a positive feedback cycle of reaching for new goals. Feeling success after success after success, each little goal takes you one step closer to living fully.

Aiming for something totally preposterous ("I want to run a marathon the week after major surgery"), unreasonable ("I want to continue working full-time, take care of my seven children without help, and keep my cancer diagnosis and chemotherapy treatments a secret from everyone"), or dependent on too many factors beyond your control ("I want to have a completely smooth course without a single setback or delay") is an invitation to frustration, disappointment, and anger. Realistic goals can keep you focused and motivated.

Tips for Reaching Your Goals

- Let others help you set healthy goals that aren't too high or low.
- Let others help you achieve your goals.
- Listen when others cheer you on.
- Let others support you through delays, setbacks, and disappointments that can be part of a successful journey.
- Invite others to celebrate your successes with you.

What are your short-term goals? Your intermediate goals?
Your long-term goals? With whom do you share your goals?

Overcoming Obstacles and Doing the Right Things

All along, I've intended to use effective action as the means to getting good care and living fully, and not as an end in and of itself. I've tried to avoid becoming like some patients who get so caught up in their survivorship that forever after their lives revolve around their illness. I want to forget about my illness. So, my goal as a patient has been to use action to help me enjoy my life outside of illness as quickly and completely as possible.

Learning about steps I could take to help my recovery and developing healthy habits suited to life after cancer have enabled me to let my illness drift into the background of my life. When I don't have to be thinking about my cancer, I don't think about it! However, when medical problems arise or decisions need to be made, I shift gears, pulling out what I know about taking proper action and trying to do the right things.

Staying unemotional when rational decisions need to be made is hard. I can't get rid of my emotions, and I can't act perfectly all the time. And, I wouldn't want to. I will always have times of consciously doing what I know is not the best course of action, such as pushing myself too hard until I feel sick instead of resting, or being cross with someone who doesn't deserve it. Healthy Survivorship includes times of making mistakes and letting my emotions get the better of me. Healthy Survivorship also includes recognizing when that is happening, forgiving myself and usually laughing at myself, and moving forward. I hope that you now recognize many of the obstacles to effective action in your life and can find ways to conquer them. The goal is to balance acting effectively with living fully.

The following are a few measures that have helped me narrow the gap between knowing the right thing to do and actually doing it. Find other measures that may help you, too.

Develop healthy goals: Define your goals. Write them down. Keep your goals in mind. Remind yourself of your goals frequently and in a variety of ways such as by hanging inspiring posters in your house, keeping a list of goals in your wallet, and talking about them with loved ones.

Minimize barriers to meeting your goals. This often takes a lot of hard work. Make an honest evaluation of the obstacles to meeting your goals, and then try to see these obstacles as challenges (and not punishment or tests): What can you do to decrease or eliminate the barrier? What can you do to get over or around the barrier? Sometimes simply modifying your environment creates a setting that gives your strengths the upper hand over your weaknesses, clears obstacles to effective action, and increases your incentive to do the right thing. For example, I use a pill-minder to increase the likelihood of taking my medicines correctly, I take my phone off the hook to increase the likelihood of getting a good nap, and I keep a basket filled with fresh fruit on the counter so it's easy to eat healthful snacks. Simple measures can make a huge difference.

Adjust your goals, as needed. When a goal is no longer a possibility, let it go and make a new goal. When a goal is still achievable but is distracting you from more pressing or more adaptive goals, refocus on healthier goals for your current situation.

Develop healthy habits and rules. Good rules and habits are your friends. As your situation changes over time, assess whether your current rules and habits are good for your current situation. In any situation where you are tempted to break a rule, stop and acknowledge the advantages of breaking the rule (there must be some upside to doing the wrong thing or you wouldn't be tempted to break the rule). Weigh those advantages against the advantages of following your rules (these advantages will almost always win out if it is a good rule). Make a list of the advantages and benefits of proper action, and the disadvantages and losses associated with not taking proper action. Read your list or think of it when tempted to abandon proper action. Following good rules leads to healthy habits. Every time you practice a way of thinking or acting, it helps you do it more naturally the next time.

Celebrate successes. No matter how small the achievement, reward yourself or celebrate in some way. Every time I flew alone to California for treatment in a clinical trial, I packed an extra $15 in my wallet. After being discharged from the hospital, I stopped by the hospital gift shop and bought myself a gift, usually a pair of earrings. These little celebrations reframed my otherwise scary and lonely cancer trips by distracting me from the reason I was going and giving me something to look forward to. Each addition to my collection of costume jewelry was a tangible reminder of my progress. Every little step forward is worthy of celebrating. Life is worth celebrating.

Develop mottoes that help you do the right thing.

Wendy's Mottoes for Taking Action

- If I can do the physically hard stuff to get well (like take my cancer treatments), surely I can do the physically easy stuff to get well and stay well (like getting exercise, eating well, resting, and reporting worrisome symptoms to my doctor).
- Doing the right thing can help me feel better while helping me get better and stay better. I don't like feeling bad, so if I can do something to keep from feeling bad, I should do it.
- My actions are one element of my healing under my complete control. Doing the right thing helps stack the odds in my favor and gives me maximum control over my life.
- I've worked too hard and sacrificed too much to stop here. A lot of other people have, too. It doesn't make sense to do the right thing only half the time.
- Doing the right thing is the best gift I could ever give to the people I love. Although I don't owe anyone anything, I *want* to show my family and friends how much I appreciate them. Doing the right thing is the most powerful and meaningful way for me to express my love.
- *Just do it!* When arguing, explaining, or cajoling fail, and when my logical or inspiring mantras aren't working, I think of the Nike directive, and I make sure I do the right thing.

What mottoes help you do the right thing?

With sound knowledge and genuine hope, you can act in ways that help you get good care and live fully. But even when you are doing everything right, you may not feel happy. Finding happiness when life is hard is the subject of the closing chapter.

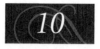

Finding Happiness in a Storm

I cannot change the wind, but I can adjust my sails.—*Source unknown*

The true voyage of discovery consists not in seeking new landscapes, but in having new eyes.—*Marcel Proust, 1871*

Illness can feel like a fierce storm, entering your life uninvited and with little warning, indiscriminatingly threatening or destroying many pleasures and hopes you hold dear. And then, during sickness and recovery, or even if the illness is behind you, the possibility that your disease might rob you of every earthly joy continues to cloud your life. I offer the notion of "happiness in a storm" as a metaphor for any happiness in the midst of difficulties accompanying your diagnosis, evaluation, treatment, recovery, or long-term survivorship. Without a doubt, illness is bad, yet, survivorship —from the time of diagnosis and for the balance of life—can include times of great joy among the hardships. You *can* find happiness.

Everyone wants happiness, but what is happiness? What is this entity so fundamental that its pursuit is one of the three basic inalienable rights of Americans, alongside life and liberty? And what's the difference between *feeling* happy and *being* happy? In overly simplistic terms, "feeling happy" is when you feel good emotionally for the moment. In contrast, "being happy" is an overarching sense of wholeness of your body, mind, and spirit that makes you glad to be alive. When you are truly happy, a sense emanates from within you that things are right in the world. Happiness in a storm is about both feeling happy and being happy when life is hard.

As a youngster, I learned that the preamble to America's Declaration of Independence doesn't guarantee happiness, only the right to *pursue* happiness. It's up to each individual to determine if and how to pursue happiness. In many circumstances, but especially when you are sick, you can't find happiness by going back to the last place you remember having it. It's not something you can buy with a dollar or nail down with a hammer. Once found, you can't hold on to happiness the way you can wrap your arms securely around a puppy and hold tight. As with your hopes, your happiness is continually redefined, re-created or rediscovered again and again as you and your circumstances evolve.

During and after illness, your challenge lies in finding happiness now, in the life you have, even though it may not be the life path you wanted, prepared for, or expected. Don't compound your misfortune by letting your pain keep you from seeing or feeling the real happiness your illness allows. It would be a tragedy if you couldn't experience the surprising little joys that spritz survivors like an ocean spray and the secrets for happiness discovered in hard times.

Happiness during treatment and recovery is often a consequence of moving through and beyond unpleasant sensations or situations. When your headache resolves, you feel happy. When a worrisome lump turns out to be nothing, you celebrate. Happiness is also tied to various emotions such as gratitude for your treatments and caregivers, or a sense of accomplishment after completing a round of treatment. Soaking in a warm bath that soothes your aching muscles or receiving a loved one's gentle kiss on your forehead can lead you to a type of happiness that is hardy like a desert flower. In contrast, walking unaided after months of physical therapy or adopting a child after years of unsuccessful fertility treatments can lead to happiness inextricably tied to preceding pain and grief, and effort and patience. These joys are like jewels that are precious not only on account of their brilliant luster but also because of the extraordinary difficulty in mining and then sculpting them. Yet another source of happiness is the possibility of so-called silver linings, good things coming out of bad times.

When I talk about my silver linings—being at home with my kids and discovering writing, having time to play my violin, and learning to cook—someone invariably asks, "Was it worth it?" They want to know if I would have chosen to develop lymphoma if I'd known ahead of time all the blessings that were going to come out of my illness. I know that they mean well and are trying to help me feel better about what's happened, but their question troubled me until I realized it made no sense. Any suggestion that my cancer was worth it (or that I might ever choose it) reflects their desire to give me a sense of control in a situation that was beyond my control. Normal people don't choose illness or injury. It just happens. Cancer happened to me. My choice lies in the life I live after cancer.

> Illness and injury happen. Illness or injury happened to you. Your choice lies in the life you live now.

Moments of feeling good can occur *despite* the storm, such as when I laughed at my husband's well-timed joke while we awaited my surgery, or when I swayed in rhythm to my favorite tune playing on the car radio and forgot about my leg pain. Precious are the joys that have arisen *because* of the storm, such as when I learned that my posttreatment scans were clear. On what was an ordinary weekday for most people, the exhilarating news of my remission made me feel like I was walking on air.

Sweet as it is, feeling happy is a limited goal because it is short-lived. The real challenge in illness is *being happy*. Discomforts, losses, and unwanted changes tend to affect your view of the world in ways that make it hard to be happy. This is especially so when you are newly diagnosed, struggling with complications or recurrence, or facing terminal disease. You can't expect to experience happiness if you have searing pain. Terror leaves no space for happiness. If the chemistry of your brain is affected in ways that block happiness, strong willpower and spiritual faith may be unable to lift your spirit in joy. Take heart; you can make changes that can help you find some happiness again, even during the tough times. This happiness derives at least partly from a life-enhancing shift in your perception of yourself and of the world around you that brings color to darkness and order to chaos. Whether it is mixed with other complex feelings or experienced as pure joy, and whether it is a fleeting feeling or an enduring way of life, happiness in a storm makes life worth fighting for.

How, exactly, do *you* find happiness in a storm? What do you need to do, think, feel, or say today in order to find happiness while you are going through your treatment or recovery, or while living with chronic disease? Chances are that opportunities for happiness are right in front of you. Maybe you've forgotten how to enjoy your favorite pastimes. You don't normally think of being able to "forget" something like working on your stamp collection or playing your guitar, but patients easily get lost in their pain, loss, and stress. In cases like these, the exercise of writing your own "personal happiness list" may be all you need to jog your memory and reintroduce delights into your daily diet. You might need to explore different ways of seeing yourself and the world around you. In doing so, you may discover *new* types of happiness waiting to be tapped, such as the happiness of sharing invigorating ideas and nascent hopes with new friends, or the happiness of knowing love in a whole new way. Happiness in a storm is never about enjoying your illness but embracing your life within the limits of your illness, and figuring out how to feel happy whenever possible.

Reading others' personal stories of happiness after illness may help guide you in refurbishing your old recipes of happiness and creating new ones. In my case, my years of observing and talking with other survivors, reading and writing about survivorship, praying alone and with friends, and much trial and error have led me to the mantras and methods that have been helping me in my pursuit of happiness. The stories that follow may help you identify obstacles to your joys and how to overcome them. Unlike following a cookie recipe, however, you can't just mimic the scenarios. Why not? The settings—the actions, attitudes, conversations, and situations—that make you happy are unique to you.

My hope is that you'll recognize something familiar in these stories, and you'll be sensitized to the many opportunities *you* have for finding and creating joy in *your* life. If my situation is completely foreign to yours, my outlook your polar opposite, and my mantras ring false, the contrast can serve to help clarify what *will* help you. For example, although my selection of Bach's partitas for violin may not excite you in the least, the idea of listening to music may lead you to play your old Beatles recordings because they always put you in a good mood! As you read this chapter, look to your future with optimism that you can find happiness again. Think about happiness and nurture your hope that it is *possible* to experience happiness in a storm.

Make a list of things and activities that used to bring you happiness. Make a list of new things that might bring you happiness.

Healthy Survivorship, Choice, and Happiness

For me, Healthy Survivorship is a necessary condition of happiness. I don't think I can be happy until I first feel confident that I am getting good care and doing what I can to heal. But Healthy Survivorship, alone, is not enough. Even when I'm confidently doing everything possible to ensure the best outcome in all spheres of my life, I still may be miserable. In addition to taking steps to get good care and live fully, I must also take steps to set the stage for happiness. I must actively seek out and create joy.

When times are tough, happiness is a choice you make and not an automatic feeling. Although developing cancer was a bad deal, I learned early on that I don't have to feel sad, scared, angry, or unhappy all the time. The knowledge-hope-action approach that has helped me find relief from both my nausea and my frustration of fatigue has also helped me find oasis after oasis of joy after cancer. First, I've obtained knowledge about the obstacles to happiness that arise during illness, and how to overcome them. Then I've nourished my belief that I can reshape my outlook and create situations to bring me happiness during treatment and recovery. Based on what I've learned and come to believe, I take steps to pursue joy. Implicit in this knowledge-hope-action approach is the fact that I *want* to feel and be happy, and that I'm willing to open my eyes to opportunities and to put in the effort. If you read no further, at least STOP for a moment and think—seriously—about your answer to the question "Do you *want* to feel happy?"

How much do you want to feel happy? How much effort are you willing to put in and how much are you willing to change in order to be happy?

Defining Your Storm

"Know thy enemy and know thy self and you will win a hundred battles" is a classic line from *The Art of War* by Sun Tzu Wu. Naturally you feel unhappy when you are sick. Have you stopped and thought in more specific terms about *why* you are unhappy? Is pain making you unhappy? Fear? Losing your hair or a body part? And what is keeping you from finding happiness again? Could your sense of uncertainty about the future or a loss of self-confidence be affecting your outlook in negative ways? Knowing your enemies—the factors that are hampering your pursuit of joy—and understanding their changing nature over time can help you.

Illness-related losses are common obstacles to joy. Grieving your losses—loss of health, friends who deserted you, opportunities, and dreams—is the only way through your pain to renewed joy. Just be sure you don't say "Good-bye, forever!" to losses that are temporary. Conversely, given the changes brought on by your illness, don't be afraid to let go of joys that no longer have a place in your life; new joys may be even greater.

Specific pleasures may be impossible in the setting of your illness. One patient couldn't go downhill skiing because his bone tumor had weakened part of his femur (thigh bone) to paper-thinness. So he took up stationary cycling until his thigh bone was completely healed and strong enough to resume skiing. For me, exercising at the local gym and work-ing in my medical practice were not options from 1990 to 1991 because my blood counts were dangerously low and I was too ill. Instead, I bought a few VCR tapes and jazzercised in my family room with a girl-friend. And, with illness keeping me from clinical medicine, I discovered the joy of writing for fellow patients. Recognizing and acknowledging your immutable losses open the path to healing grief. Then you can search for short-term alternatives to temporary losses and for different ways to achieve a sense of pleasure after permanent losses.

Old pleasures may be possible only after making some changes. In 1993, I was at my lowest point emotionally. While dealing with cancer recurrences and taking medications that affected my brain, I couldn't listen to my favorite classical music. Mozart's lilting sonatinas and Beethoven's *Ode to Joy* dragged me down. The musical notes were cer-tainly the same as always, and my hearing was fine. The mood-altering side effects of my multiple medications made happiness almost impossi-ble. I spoke to my physicians, who adjusted my medications. Then I could recapture the joy of music. If you yearn to enjoy certain activities but obstacles keep holding you back, get help resolving fixable problems and adjusting to irreversible ones. Save yourself time and energy by talk-ing with a friend or counselor who can help you sort through the com-plex reasons why you are finding joy elusive.

Who can help you identify and overcome the physical, emotional, and practical obstacles to enjoying pleasurable situa-tions and activities? Who can help you understand and grieve your losses? Who can support you as you let go of past pleasures?

Humor

I grew up in a family where jokes and puns peppered dinnertime conver-sations and were used routinely to diffuse tensions and to buoy one another in uncomfortable situations. Looking for something to laugh at is an ingrained reflex that has helped me relieve the seriousness of my ill-ness and stay in touch with the joyful world. More than just helping me get through treatment and recovery, humor helps me find happiness in tough times. Humor is highly personal and, in usual circumstances, spontaneous. Nobody can force you to see humor in an awful situation any more than someone can force you to love someone you find repul-sive. But that doesn't mean that you can't take steps to benefit from the healing power of your own style of humor when the last thing you feel like doing is smiling.

Few things are as reliably heartening as retelling an inside family joke or comical episode. Harpham lore includes the story of my introductory meeting with my Canadian in-laws. Over appetizers, they were exchang-ing jokes. Taking the plunge, I nervously pitched a setup question, "How do you know if you have a thousand pounds of pickles under your bed?" They all looked at Ted's new girlfriend—me—and before anyone could attempt an answer I started to giggle. Within seconds, I was laughing uncontrollably and had to leave the living room. After a minute or two, I headed back to deliver the punch line, but as soon as I saw them I broke up laughing and had to turn around and leave. This back and forth went on for five minutes until—picture this: I dashed by the entryway to the living room, blurting out "Because you are closer to the ceiling!" From the hallway, I watched my future in-laws, bewildered, exchange glances all around before erupting together in laughter. Ever since, when a family situation is begging for comic relief, someone might ask, "Pickle, any-one?" Any reference to the "P word" has been good medicine when I've been dealing with the mix of emotions surrounding the diagnostic and follow-up tests and the repeated courses of my cancer treatments. My pathetically unfunny pickle joke has been one way for me to begin to regain a sense of control in otherwise overwhelming circumstances.

Humor pokes fun at difficult or embarrassing topics, which is why sex, money, parenting, and politics are popular topics of stand-up comedy. Joking about these other serious topics may distract you from your cur-rent problems and keep you involved in the healthy world that includes other troubles. It also can help keep your medical challenges in perspec-tive (yours are not the only problems in the world). If you don't have the energy or creativity right now to make jokes or puns, you can read comics and humorous books, watch funny shows and movies, or hang around people who make you laugh. If you can't imagine laughing now (or ever again), I urge you to go to a support group meeting where people in situations similar to yours enjoy socializing and laughing together in a setting where illness is normal and life goes on.

We are talking about the *pursuit* of happiness. Don't just sit there waiting to feel happy. You might have to relearn how to laugh, just as you'd have to relearn how to walk or eat soup with a spoon if illness impaired your ability to do these things that used to come naturally. Even if at first you feel self-conscious, resentful, or pessimistic, keep trying. With time, you'll tap into your own personal blend of humor that helps you through tough times. So, go out and tickle your funny bone or have someone tickle it for you.

Soon after I was diagnosed, I borrowed *Candid Camera* videos that are sent free of charge to patients as part of Allen Funt's nonprofit foundation's Laughter Therapy program. Even though I was on the verge of feeling overwhelmed with fear and grief, and even though I had the surreal sense that I was mechanically humoring myself with videos, it worked! I couldn't help but laugh at some of the antics. Each smile or giggle made me feel a bit more normal and in control. When I was laughing, I couldn't be crying, which felt good, too.

Every evening throughout the months of my initial chemotherapy my husband and I escaped into fantasy by watching tapes of *Star Trek*. Find something that you enjoy. One man living with painful multiple myeloma, a type of bone cancer, enthusiastically followed the Texas Rangers baseball games. Throughout the spring and summer, he enjoyed the pregame anticipation, game-time excitement, and inning-by-inning rehashing after the game. Baseball was his life raft, keeping him afloat from one weekend to the next. Everyone has *something* that makes him or her feel happy. Look for ways to forget about serious matters for a moment or two and lose yourself in sports, fantasy, literature, movies, music, art, or something else you find entertaining. Pleasure recharges your batteries when going through hard times, so find things to smile and laugh about.

You could laugh at your medical problems because illness is funny.

Well, no, not really. Serious illness is never funny. But it can give rise to amusing situations. I've enjoyed a lot of laugh mileage out of the incident when a nurse came into my hospital room to check my vital signs while my regular nurse was on lunch break. I was fully dressed, sitting in a chair, working on my laptop computer with my IV pole unintentionally camouflaged between me and the wall. My husband was asleep on the bed. The young nurse looked at me, then at Ted, then back at me, and asked, "Uh, who is the patient?"

A seventy-ish-year-old friend, Aphy, told me her humorous story of going to the clinic one day for her routine blood work. When the medical assistant reached to take her blood pressure, Aphy pulled back, saying, "No, you can't use this arm. I've had a mastectomy." The young woman looked at Aphy rather strangely and asked, "You've had a *vasectomy*?" "No, not vasectomy. Mastectomy!" The technician clearly doubted the correction, mumbling, "These days, who knows?"

Aphy's story is especially instructive. When I first e-mailed her and asked if she might have a fun story to share, she responded immediately with a despondent e-mail message that read, "Nothing is going right, Wendy, and I just can't think of anything happy or funny right now." I immediately sent her a reply, telling her, "I understand. Please forget about my request." I ended my message with a few words of comfort and hope. Later that evening, I had a new message from Aphy in my e-mail in-box. She first told me her mastectomy-vasectomy story. Then she wrote, "Wendy, I haven't thought of this incident since it happened. Remembering and e-mailing it to you made me smile for the first time in days. Thanks!" All I had done was ask "Can you think of something funny?" Without her even trying, the memory emerged, lifting her from desolation. As you go through the rigmarole of treatment and recovery, keep your eyes open for amusing situations that can lift your spirits. Multiply the pleasure by sharing your stories. Some medical situations are innately funny, and others are so because you respond in a way that makes the situation amusing. My first recurrence was diagnosed on May 30, 1992. Needless to say, that became a personal date of infamy. Exactly one year later, on May 30, 1993, after radiation and interferon treatments had put my cancer back into remission, I was scheduled for my routine follow-up. I had no obvious signs of cancer, so I was expecting a good checkup. But my scans revealed recurrent disease. While still in shock from the news after meeting with my oncologist, my husband and I met with my internist in her office. With a straight face, I said, "I've consolidated my recurrence dates. By having this recurrence on the same date as my last one, I won't have too many bad-news anniversaries!" Then I giggled and smiled at Ted. My internist studied me, assessing if I was in denial. Believe me, I was well aware of the seriousness of my situation. My spontaneous joke, albeit a typically Wendy stupid one, helped me feel less frightened and gave me back a sense of control. Over the next few days, while sharing the news of my recurrence with family and friends, I could temper *their* distress by teasing about the convenience of scheduling my recurrence for May 30.

Making jokes about painful aspects of my survivorship has been an effective tool for giving me a sense of command over much of the unavoidable stress and loss. Humor has helped me present difficult problems to my children in ways that indicate my desire to accept unwanted change and loss, and move forward with optimism. For instance, when I was going through chemotherapy, my family often played off of the classic vaudeville repartee in which a woman insults W. C. Fields, saying "Sir, you are drunk!" and W. C. Fields responds, "Madam, you are ugly. And I'll be sober in the morning!" (Ted would say to me, "You are more bald than me!" Our children and I would look at Ted's receding hairline while I'd respond, "Yeah, but after the chemo is done, *my* hair is growing back!" Then I'd wink at the kids as if Ted were a real loser and I had the upper hand.) On so many levels this brief comedy routine was healing for my family: reminding everyone that my baldness was temporary; feeling power over the baldness by joking about it; suggesting a sense of unity between Ted and me; adding a layer of levity to an unwanted change; and encouraging my children to adjust to the change by laughing at it.

Humor helped me nourish more long-lasting happiness, too, by giving helpful clues as to what was bothering me or making me sad, and by providing entry into discussions about serious issues. Bringing them out in the open helped me accept and adjust to unwanted changes. For instance, I remember the time I had bruises on my arms from the repeated needle sticks and a large bandage on my neck from a recent biopsy. While walking out of the bedroom, I accidentally bumped into the corner of my night-stand and cried out to Ted, "Oh no! I'm going to get a black-and-blue mark, and my body won't be perfect anymore!" We literally fell to the ground laughing. After a series of leg-crossing, tear-wiping laughing spells, we finally settled down and enjoyed that pleasant posthysteria exhaustion.

> To laugh at what threatens you is to diminish its power to frighten.
> To laugh at what saddens you is to lighten the load of your grief.
> To laugh at yourself and your situation is to regain control over your life.

It gave us an opening to share our sadness over the physical changes and losses of my illness, and encouraged us to accept them and move forward with hope. As I write this, I can still hear in my head Ted's laugh from all those years ago, and the memory is making me smile. I suspect this episode was one of those "You had to be there" moments. Maybe you'd *never* be able to laugh at bumping into a table. That's okay, too. The message is that when the timing is right, actively choosing to laugh at some of the hard stuff gives you a way to find a bit of happiness in otherwise sad circumstances. As we say in my house, "A no-hair day is better than a bad-hair day." And "No nodes is good nodes!" By helping you face and tame your fears, accept and adjust to losses, and work your way through problems, humor intended to help you feel happy for a moment or two can lead to discussions and changes that help you to become happy.

What family jokes or stories make you smile? What occurrences or situations can you poke fun at or turn into a joke?

Pleasure

Your senses are always ready and waiting to transport pleasurable signals to your brain, where they can affect it in ways that make it easier to feel good right now. You can facilitate pleasure by making the effort to visit or create sensual environments of sights, sounds, smells, tastes, and textures that elicit your sense of peacefulness, inspiration, or delight. Maybe you enjoy sitting on a bench in a nearby park, or fingering all the new gizmos at the local hardware store, or listening to live music by local artists at a nearby cafe. Think of those special places and spaces where you feel good, and make an effort to go there.

Create "feel-good" spaces in your home, too. Set up a table or desk with your favorite games, reading material, or equipment for writing letters, painting watercolors, putting ships in bottles, or whatever else you like to do. Take an exotic minivacation without leaving home by soaking in a bubble bath or by looking through picture albums that revive happy memories. Visit your "feel-good" spaces even when you still have errands waiting (as long as they aren't urgent). Make your pursuit of happiness one of your top priorities each day alongside ensuring good nutrition, regular exercise, and restorative sleep.

Decorate your home in a way that encourages peacefulness, contentment, and joy. I painted the walls of my study bright rose and the doors grape purple! Most people who visit my study laugh at me or roll their eyes ("What was she thinking?"). It's not their room; it's mine. Pink and purple make me feel energized and happy. Even if your current "home" is an isolation room in a hospital, you can find ways to transform this living space into a healing place.

Tips for Creating Healing Spaces

- Surround yourself with the colors that make you feel good. Wall hangings, mobiles, sun catchers, stained-glass windows, shelf knick-knacks, your bedding, and your clothing should reflect colors that make you smile.
- Accent your room with life-affirming plants. If you can't be around live foliage because your immune system is suppressed, or if caring for houseplants is not your thing, fool your senses by creating an atmosphere of perennial springtime with realistic-looking silk flowers.
- Fill the air with mood-lifting sounds by playing music or recorded nature sounds, hanging wind chimes, or setting up a tabletop water-fountain rock garden.

- Use pleasing perfumes or aftershave, body wash, body lotions, or shampoo. Sleep in freshly washed sheets, pillowcases, and blankets. Burn fragrant candles.
- Stimulate your senses by wearing clothing with cozy textures such as soft cotton, velvet or velour, satin, or corduroy. Make up your bed with soothing sheets and pillows. Keep a comfort object within reach—a smooth stone for rubbing, a soft stuffed animal for hugging, a cat curled up on your lap for stroking, or a dog asleep at your feet for petting.
- Adjust your lighting to create a peaceful or happy mood.
- Hang pictures or posters to help you remember the places you enjoy and the important people in your life.
- Display inspirational sayings and symbols on wall hangings, desktop plaques, and your clothing. Keep close at hand uplifting books that touch your heart, and get in the habit of reading them regularly.

Where can you go for a "happiness break"? What activities that make you happy can you still do? What can you do to create a happy living space?

Giving

"To give is to receive." This aphorism is no more poignant and powerful than when you are sick and feel that all you do is take, take, take. The stress of getting through my initial chemotherapy was made more difficult by the added demands of my three young kids. In a few important ways, however, being forced to shift from Wendy-patient to Wendy-mom helped me through this time. Whether reading to my kids or tending to their skinned knees, the acts of mothering transported me outside my self-centered and depressing world of cancer by highlighting and exercising parts of me that were still healthy and strong. When I wasn't too tired or sick, giving to my children helped me to feel whole and find happiness.

As long as you are not overextending yourself by reaching out to someone else, the combination of distraction from illness, connection to others, and sense of meaning eases the stress of your illness and elicits joyful feelings. Engaging in acts of giving can reduce any lingering anger or frustration with your losses. When thinking of others' needs, you are distracting yourself from your own troubles, numbing your pain, and gaining a sense of purpose in otherwise painful times.

Helping others doesn't just help you feel better; it may actually help you get better. Studies have shown that healthy elderly people who give support to friends and relatives show improvement in their quality and length of life compared to those of comparable health who don't reach out to help others. Other studies have indicated that helping others is associated with improved immune functioning, fewer colds and headaches, and relief from pain and insomnia. Helping is good for your health.

This notion of healing through giving helped me even before I was able to give anything to anyone. A few days after my original diagnosis, my children's pediatrician asked Clare, a young mom, to call me. Clare had been through a bone-marrow transplant a couple of years earlier. This angel talked with me for an hour or so, all the while answering my questions and assuring me that I could and would raise my kids while going through treatment. As our conversation wound down and I expressed appreciation, she said, "You can thank me by helping someone else when you are better."

Her words touched a chord: "No matter what I'm going through, I am learning something that might help someone else down the line." By linking my pain to potentially valuable lessons, she gave me confidence that I would survive to use what I was learning now to help someone later. The hard times were still painful, but, in having meaning, they felt less so. I didn't wait long before tasting the special joy of giving to other survivors. When I was still a "newbie" at chemo, a fashionable woman in my doctor's reception room started up a conversation by complimenting my head scarf. Soon I was offering her a tip about getting a short haircut before her hair fell out. Imagine how good I felt to see her eyes, wide with fear when we'd started talking, crinkle in the corners with the glint of someone with a job to do.

Helping others sends a message that is loud and clear: "I am not at rock bottom! I still have something to offer." You may be wondering what you could give or how you could possibly give anything when you feel so needy yourself. Opportunities always exist for giving to others. Many members of my cancer support group made themselves available to talk on the phone to newly diagnosed patients. Still others spent time composing poems or writing articles for survivorship newsletters or magazines, helping with fund-raisers, or baking goodies for our cancer-support-group meetings.

You are not obligated or expected to help other patients at any phase of your survivorship. Between your doctor visits and treatments, you may do best to avoid dealing with your illness in any other context. Or, if you are involved in helping patients now, you are not obligated to continue these efforts indefinitely. For many survivors, a time comes when the surest path to happiness is to walk away from reminders of illness. Don't be trapped in the difficult sides of survivorship. Just because you are *able* to help other patients doesn't mean you should. The best gift you can give yourself and your loved ones is doing whatever it takes for you to get better and feel better. If your best course of action is to avoid patients and hospitals, you help everyone by respecting that. Use your experience and insights to help other patients only if doing so makes you feel strong, inspired, confident, fulfilled, or happy.

Another approach is to pursue one of the infinite numbers of giving opportunities that have nothing to do with illness. Through the ups and downs of the course of his rocky treatment, one man in my support group continued his long-standing volunteer work holding premature babies at the county hospital. Another patient helped her daughter address wedding invitations and served as a sounding board for a friend who was considering a job change. One chronically bedridden patient, too weak to write a note, offered prayers for individuals who she was told needed them. In all but the direst circumstances you can give in some way, even if only by making the effort to articulate heartfelt appreciation to those who are caring for you. As long as you are not jeopardizing your health, reach out to someone else and see if helping others helps you.

Even when focusing your energies away from the settings of illness, you can reap the joy of inspiring other patients. Much has been made of cyclist Lance Armstrong's comeback after being cured of widespread testicular cancer. Justifiably so. He broke all records in 2004 by winning the 2,000-mile Tour de France for the sixth time in a row after recovering from cancer treatments that included brain surgery and intensive chemotherapy. Almost every time I mount the StairMaster at my local gym I think of Lance and say to myself, "If he can train for hours every day in the mountains, surely I can work out in this air-conditioned gym for forty-five minutes." Jeff Berman of the *New York Times* wrote of Lance in July 2003, "He is not only an amazing athlete with an inspirational story; he is proof of something very important and very exciting: Cancer is not a death sentence, and people can come back from it even stronger." And for many of you, long-term survivorship in superior physical health is possible. Those of you with ongoing physical losses or limitations can come back stronger in other ways—your spirit, outlook, sense of purpose, and joyfulness.

The mistake is to assume that you have to do something grand to inspire someone else. Actually, you don't have to run a marathon or establish a new philanthropic foundation. Being a patient opens opportunities for you to save lives with the smallest of acts. How? Since everyone becomes a patient someday, your words and actions are affecting people who fear or deny the possibility of getting sick themselves, as well as those who are dealing with illness right now. If, during treatment, you eat breakfast in the morning and go to a movie at night you are sending a message that there is life after illness. If you get through treatment-related complications, you teach others that setbacks can occur on the path to a good outcome. If you let people know that you are having a rough time emotionally but you are getting support, you are showing people that it is not shameful to struggle, and that accepting help is a good thing.

My friend Scotty e-mailed to all his friends and family a photo his wife took of him in his sunglasses, wearing a Hawaiian lei around his neck and holding a large cup adorned with one of those silly little paper umbrellas. Was he trying to make us jealous of his holiday at a beachfront resort? Hardly. Scotty was sitting in a hospital-issue recliner, hooked up to three bags of intravenous medicines, enjoying a little goofy fun as he awaited his stem-cell transplant. For all Scotty knows, someday the memory of this joyful picture may be the reason why someone else decides to have a lump checked out immediately instead of delaying, or feels hopeful when entering a hospital! The Talmud, an ancient collection of Jewish laws and traditions, teaches that if you save one life you save a world. Without your even realizing it and without your even making a conscious effort to make a difference, your experiences as a patient may save a world one day.

Talk with friends or a counselor and make a list of opportunities to reach out. Check with your doctors that these activities are okay.

Taking the Road Not Taken Before

As a high-school student I couldn't imagine going two whole days in a row without playing my violin. However, I also knew that I'd retire my violin after I hung out my doctor's shingle, at least until I was done raising my family. For this is the nature of life: When you come to a fork in the road, every time you choose to do *this* or go *here*, you also are choosing *not* to do *that* or go *there*. This necessary loss can be painful, as Robert Frost acknowledges with the phrase "And sorry I could not travel both," in "The Road Not Taken," his poem about two roads diverging in a yellow wood.

In 1983 my dream of practicing medicine became reality when I opened my own office and began what was to be a lifetime of caring for patients. "And sorry I could not travel both"—unread books, unwritten letters, and unplayed music were accepted as part of the price of doing what I wanted to do. In 1990, a week or two after being diagnosed with cancer, I found myself suddenly with too much time on my hands and was feeling lost. So I dusted off my violin case, took out my violin, tightened the strings and bow, and began playing music again. I've been playing on and off ever since.

I do believe I would have felt happy and fulfilled had I stayed healthy and continued caring for my patients until I retired at eighty years old. But in taking the road not taken earlier—in leaving clinical medicine behind and embracing the life of a writer—I've been able to savor many of the joys I willingly sacrificed when I decided to become a physician: reading books on religion and philosophy, writing lengthy e-mails and letters, cheering at my daughters' volleyball games during the day, and playing the violin with my son at night. Unexpectedly, I've been able to travel both roads.

Sometimes you continue down a path because it is the right path for you, and the only reason you'd ever change course is because your chosen path becomes impossible. Other times you continue down a path because you don't realize that another might be better. Or you suspect you would be better off elsewhere, but you can't imagine finding the guts or the momentum needed to leave something familiar and comfortable.

Illness can give you a fresh start by causing a major shake-up in your normal routines, clearing your mind and heart of emotional obstacles that are keeping you in a rut. This reminds me of times when I have a glitch in my computer program. Sometimes I can fix it, but usually the best course of action is to turn off my machine and boot up again. Somehow, shutting down the system for a minute clears the problems and allows me to move forward. A diagnosis of serious disease

> Happiness in a storm is seeing the possibilities that were always there and finding the courage and strength needed to go down a better path.

reboots your outlook by causing you to experience a shift in your priorities, perception of risk, and sense of purpose. It is never too late to change direction and take the road not taken before.

It is not just you who may be taking a new road but also the important people in your life. Before my diagnosis, my husband worked at home when he wasn't teaching college classes. He cared for our little ones until I got home from work, at which time he'd put a home-cooked dinner on the table for the family. All that changed when I got sick and became a writer. Now Ted leaves home early in the morning so that I can have the house to write and rest. Now I make dinner. If Ted wanted to be happy after my cancer, his routines and expectations had to change when my path changed. It is not a matter of our new lives being better or worse, although Ted will tell you that I make a tasty sesame chicken dinner. What matters is that we both found ways to be happy by letting go of the routines that we'd expected, planned for, and gotten used to during the early years of our marriage.

The unwanted changes prompted by your illness may open opportunities to do things differently. This is your chance to find new ways to feel happy and be happy. Stories abound of survivors who brave skydiving or horseback riding for the first time, write the book they've been threatening to write for decades, or renew vows with a loved one. Through illness, they see how to make some long-standing dreams come true and find the courage to do it.

You may find new ways to be happy if you see your illness as a fork in the road, offering you an opportunity to choose a different path. Maybe your new direction involves something as dramatic as a career change that satisfies a lifelong passion or the repair of a ravaged relationship lost for years in bitter silence. The change in direction may be more gradual and subtle. You may choose to walk with equanimity where there once was impatience, compassion where there once was indifference, or humor where there was once only seriousness. The alteration in your course may be invisible to the casual observer yet change your life in profound ways. You may choose gratitude instead of expectation and faith where there was none. Illness can be an opportunity to take the road not taken before. And that makes all the difference.

> Illness and injury open opportunities to find new ways to feel happy and be happy.

What are your choices now regarding your career? Your closest relationships? Your friendships? How much leisure time do you have, and how do you spend it? How do you spend your money? Are your priorities and outlook still the same after illness?

Faith

People often say, "You won't find an atheist in a foxhole." I'm not so sure. I've known people who didn't believe in God or any Supreme Being before they faced life-threatening illness or injury and who continued to feel the same way afterward. What I am sure of, though, is that I won't find someone in a foxhole whose belief system remains untested.

Everyone has a belief system because people are spiritual beings. By this, I mean that people develop unique beliefs about themselves and the universe that help them live with awareness of their mortality and with the many mysteries of life. If suddenly your life feels threatened in the foxhole of a hospital bed, it is natural that issues of spirituality arise. Even if your prognosis is excellent, you are facing your mortality in a new way. Being diagnosed with serious disease tests your beliefs about God, the meaning of life, and, most specifically, the purpose of *your* life.

Tested beliefs are strong beliefs.

Welcoming an exploration of your spirituality can, in the long run, help you deal with the uncertainty, pain, loss, and unfairness inherent in survivorship and thus diminish anger, confusion, frustration, and feelings of guilt or shame. In finding out what you really believe—*whatever* you believe—you grow more confident of your belief system, and this confidence can bring you joy.

After I left home for college and medical school, I attended Sabbath services now and then and observed many holidays. For the most part, however, I satisfied my need for spirituality not through organized religion or personal prayer but through heartfelt efforts to learn the science of medicine and the art of healing. During the weeks after my cancer diagnosis, I became preoccupied with existential questions. I *had* to know if I believed in God and, if so, if God could hear me. My rabbi came to my home regularly to pray and study with me. Over the next few years of cancer recurrences and various treatments, mystical experiences touched my soul and nourished my trust in a universal order beyond my farthest-stretched imagination.

My spiritual life took a dramatic turn one sizzling Texas day in mid-June of 1992 when I was strapped onto an icy-cold table in a chilly room, my head held motionless by a custom-made plastic mesh mask and the rest of me immobilized by fear—fear of imminent radiation therapy, fear of my lymphoma, and fear of pain and death. The technician shut the heavy lead door, leaving me the only living creature in the room. The machine's light focused on my neck and chest, and a buzz sounded. Without realizing what

I was doing, I started chanting in my head the familiar Hebrew words of the ancient central prayer of Judaism. The words of the Shema were rote, but the prayerfulness behind them was foreign and emanated from an unfamiliar part of me. I believe it came from my soul. What struck me was not the newfound spirituality of my fervent praying but that I felt heard. Mine was the only heartbeat in that radiation suite, but I was not alone. With all earthly distractions silenced, I experienced an indescribable sense of spiritual company in my physical aloneness. Once introduced to this awareness, I've been able to tap into it ever since. It brings me peace and strength whenever needed. Like Job, I don't *know* if I connected with God in that radiation suite, not the way I know if I'm hungry or I know that two plus two equals four. I have *faith*, and it's a faith that has made my life happier.

Throughout my survivorship I've experienced silences that have fostered my spiritual growth. Timeless sanctuaries for intense soul-searching and prayer took form within the rings of CT scanners, on the gurneys of the hospital emergency and operating rooms, and under the bright lights of the examination rooms. The mind-altering effects of middle-of-the-night wakefulness are familiar to almost anyone who has been through a life crisis. When I can't fall back asleep, accepting the sleeplessness creates an opportunity to deepen my faith.

People may come to you with the expectation that you possess deep insights about life and death. Of course, disease does not automatically endow you with a direct line to God or an answer book to great questions. What your illness may do, however, is stimulate you to tackle these questions. It can affect your outlook—some cancer survivors call their changed perspective "cancer vision"—so that introspection and soul-searching lead to answers that work for you. As with almost everything else you accomplish after your diagnosis, finding your answers to spiritual questions may require time, effort, and patience.

Opening yourself to the spiritual opportunities of your illness may bring you joy but also leaves you vulnerable. Exploring your spirituality can be unsettling even under the best of circumstances. Enlist the support of people who love you and understand you. And beware the danger of others pushing their beliefs on you, making you feel guilty or responsible for your illness or unhappiness if you don't share their spiritual faith.

If faith were the cure-all some claim it to be, how do you explain the fact that popes and babies get sick? Genuine personal faith is healing when it helps you get good care and live fully.

In facing your mortality you may discover faith for the first time. You may learn how to pray, or you may join religious services and study groups. If you had religious faith before your illness, you may reinforce your long-standing beliefs and enjoy the comfort, strength, direction, and hope that come from *tested* faith. Another possibility is that you join the patients who abandon their professed religion, finding it empty. Instead you may enjoy a new belief system and a different way to express your spirituality, one that feels more genuine and comforting. It is also possible that you'll hold on to old beliefs but only after taking them in a different direction. Whatever you believe, tested beliefs are strong beliefs that can create a satisfying sense of wholeness that leads to happiness.

*Has illness awakened your faith in religion or a philosophy?
Can you use your belief system to help support you during
this time?*

Gratitude

An attitude of gratitude creates blessings.—*Sir John Templeton*

Sir John Templeton, the famed businessman and philanthropist, teaches that gratitude can shape your life in positive ways. Illness offers many opportunities to feel gratitude, a sense of thankfulness and appreciation. Spontaneous gratitude is thankfulness that happens naturally. This effortless type of gratitude arises when patients receive good news, such as when Clare learned that her brother was a near-perfect match for her needed bone-marrow transplant and when I got through my final round of treatment smoothly. Anytime a patient hears those welcomed words, "Your disease responded well, and you are done with treatment," spontaneous gratitude bursts forth like a rainbow in a sun shower.

Conscious gratitude, in contrast to spontaneous gratitude, is thankfulness that takes effort. To experience conscious gratitude, you have to choose to focus on what's right, good, and pleasingly plentiful. It's easy to see how conscious gratitude can enhance your life if your treatments are behind you and your disease is cured, but what if you are in the middle of a rocky course of treatment and your future is uncertain? With all the losses associated with your illness—loss of comfort and confidence in the future, to name just two—why would you choose to feel grateful now? And, grateful for what?

Practicing gratitude can bring you happiness in the shadow of your loss and pain. How? Ralph Waldo Emerson wrote, "For every minute you are angry you lose sixty seconds of happiness." After an appallingly delayed diagnosis, a patient stuck in anger toward his prior physician can't feel the same happiness as a patient who feels gratitude for the competence and caring of his new doctor. A patient who feels bitter about the hardships of treatment can't feel the same happiness as a patient who focuses on gratitude for the opportunity to receive treatment. Gratitude helps dissolve not only anger but also disappointment, frustration, jealousy, and self-consciousness that can get in the way of happiness. Gratitude focuses your attention on your strengths and the big and little pleasures available to you today. Thus, gratitude can give you fortitude and optimism for weathering tough treatments, and this confidence decreases negative emotions that are obstructing joy.

Take a few minutes to remind yourself of all the things that are right in your world—all the medical complications that could have happened but didn't, all the possibilities for improvement that are still open to you, and all the love and caring surrounding you. When you eat, gratitude helps you enjoy nourishing your body even if food tastes like cardboard. When you read, thankfulness encourages you to leave illness behind and lose yourself in the written word. If you can walk, your appreciation for your mobility and independence may lead you to walk more, which helps your conditioning, which helps you feel better, which helps you feel happier. Your gratitude for the companionship of friends and family generates a balm of love. During treatment and recovery, as the Hausa people of Nigeria say, "Give thanks for a little and you will find a lot."

When I was ten, I went on an Independence Day march with my classmates. Halfway through I got a pebble in my shoe and was forced to walk a few blocks before I could stop and remove it. I was struck by how my discomfort caused me to value the simple pleasure of walking without foot pain. In a similar way, my illness has taught me to appreciate the everyday pleasures of feeling hungry before a meal and sleeping through the night. Unlike the gratitude that faded soon after removing the pebble from my shoe when I was a kid, my gratitude toward my body is ingrained because the discomforts during my initial treatments were harsh and prolonged, and residual scars remind me of them daily. Until I can get rid of the ache in my right leg and my afternoon fatigue, I'll use them to make my life happier. How? By letting them remind me of how much healthier and more comfortable I am today than when I was diagnosed. By keeping me aware of all that might have been lost had the treatments not worked. Cancer teaches me gratitude, and gratitude brings me joy.

Conscious gratitude doesn't always come easily. It took years of introspection, prayer, and counseling for me to transform my unavoidable discomforts from a source of anxiety ("Is my cancer coming back?") and sadness ("I'm not the same as I was before. I can't do this or that anymore") to one of heightened joy. I suspect that had I not resisted my unavoidable losses, and had I learned sooner to be accepting and grateful for residual discomforts, I might have more easily used them to help me find happiness.

A great challenge for me was figuring out how to transform my heightened sense of uncertainty from a source of fear to one of joy. The problem was that after my cancer diagnosis, I knew—really knew, in a way that I think might be impossible without personally facing a life crisis—that all comfort and routine can dissolve in an instant. A worrisome headache, lump, or change in a mole could propel me on another medical roller-coaster ride. For the first few years of my survivorship, my heightened sense of vulnerability caused me great distress and made it hard for me to feel or be happy, even when my medical condition was on the upswing. How could I feel happy today knowing that my health might be worse tomorrow?

Some patients achieve Healthy Survivorship by denying life's uncertainty, and that works well for them. Not for me. So my challenge became figuring out how to turn the same hyperawareness that used to *steal* my joy into a force that would *enhance* my joy. Consciously choosing to be grateful for life's uncertainty has changed my perception of all I have in positive ways. Clichéd but absolutely true, the only thing that is certain is today, this minute, this moment right now. *This* is it. Cancer gave me today, every day, in a way I'd never known before. Since I no longer take much of *anything* for granted, everything has an added element of happy surprise—I made it to see this, do that, stay here, and go there! The ordinary has become marvelous. Even unpleasant times are less painful, for they are proof that I am still here.

> Illness and injury encourage you to know both the fragility and the hopes of life, and with this knowledge to live most fully.

Illness and injury encourage you to know both the fragility and the hopes of life, and with this knowledge to live most fully. When you are happy, you can be grateful to be happy. Conversely, when you live with gratitude, you can find happiness more easily *because* you are grateful. Nurture gratitude and open your eyes, mind, and heart to joy.

Make a list of all the things for which you are grateful. How is your body serving you well? Who is on your side, caring for and about you? What is right in the world?

Relationships

Why are dramatic movies, books, and television soap operas so engaging? Think about how many movies and books feature a character suffering from an illness that prompts profound and poetic dialogue. Writers know that in the setting of serious illness, true character is exposed, central issues are clarified, and relationships take on a level of intensity that is pleasurable even when the circumstances are horrific. Why is that? Because these relationships feel more *real*. Your illness—as unwanted as it is—can serve as the backdrop to the most authentic and satisfying relationships you've ever experienced.

From the moment my IV pole and I entered the radiology reception area and I settled myself in one of the seats set in a wide circle of chairs for my first support-group meeting, I became part of a living tableau of the greatest potential of human interaction. Beginning with the genial welcomes and introductions, the conversation cut through all the crap—the politics, self-interest, distractions, superficiality, insincerity, or apathy that characterizes so many social and professional interactions. Everyone had only two things in mind: helping each other and helping ourselves. In the midst of great pain, I witnessed a seamless and endless blend of humor, altruism, resilience, patience, courage, and hope. One young mother in remission offered to adopt the baby of a single mom in treatment who was in agony over "what if?" When a distressed patient needed time to compose his thoughts, the group waited patiently as if each of us had all the time in the world and nothing on our minds at that moment except his needs.

My vulnerability and need for help opened the door to a new dimension of relating to others, including friends and loved ones. I sometimes joke that my cancer diagnosis was like an invitation to the dress rehearsal for my funeral. People shared intimate thoughts that are usually reserved for eulogies. Their expression of feelings in conversations and wordless gestures has been the closest thing to true love I can imagine. My weakness and my willingness to accept help made it possible for friends and family members to do more than just tell me they loved me; seeing me at my ugliest, literally and figuratively, they could show me they loved me. Happiness in a storm is knowing I'm loved in a way I couldn't know before and carrying others' love with me into doctor's reception rooms and oncology radiation suites and everywhere else I go.

What is striking is how many friends and colleagues *did* find ways to reach out with cards and letters, gifts, donations to cancer organizations, phone calls, and meals delivered to my home. My happiness in my storm has included surprise gifts: my next-door neighbor mowing our lawn while I was hospitalized and a trio of neighborhood moms planting my spring garden for me. For the long months of my initial treatments, people baby-sat my children and took them on outings, showing overwhelming caring and selflessness toward me and my family. And in the years of recurrences that followed, friends and colleagues continued to be supportive when I needed them. My perception of people, in general, and of certain friends and family members, in particular, has been forever changed in positive ways. Killers, thieves, and terrorists may monopolize newspaper headlines, but I know that it is the millions of individuals who help others and quietly go about their unheralded lives who form the true fabric underlying society.

> Happiness in a storm is knowing you are loved in ways you couldn't know before and carrying others' love with you everywhere you go.

Not all relationships were enhanced, mind you. I was surprised and distressed when supposed friends said or did hurtful things or withdrew from me, such as the time I entered a crowded elevator and saw a white-coated colleague quickly drop his gaze and then stare at his shoes throughout our ride up to the floor of my oncologist's office. He and others were the exceptions, though. I believe they simply didn't know how to deal with me or were dealing with their own unresolved issues about illness and mortality. Other friends and family chose to avoid saying anything at all rather than risk saying the wrong thing. On a practical level, my illness has been a filter that has shown me who my friends are. I had to let the disappointments go and not waste my time and energy worrying about them.

I also had to be willing to walk away from situations and people who were dragging me down. In short order, I learned to steer clear of people who could only look at me with pitying eyes or who devoured every detail of my medical treatments but couldn't talk about anything else with me. I became adroit at recognizing people who insisted on sharing medical horror stories or who made sport of doctor bashing, and I avoided these people like the plague. Some relationships faded away not because of any problems or tensions but because I'd moved on. For instance, I stopped attending a support group after four rewarding years because it just wasn't what I needed anymore.

In your search for happiness, pay attention to all the love and caring that come your way. Display the gifts and cards where they can remind you that people care about you. Buy a simple notebook and set it out as a "guest book" for people to sign when they visit you. At least once a day, take a moment to look at the tangible evidence of your value to others. Whether you are relating to someone via a support-group meeting, a healing prayer circle, a lunch date with a friend, or a telephone call with a loved one, embrace the authenticity nourished by your illness. Remember and hold on to the richness of your relationships, a joy that can persist long after the threat of your illness fades away.

Be ready to move on if and when the time is right for you. Meaningful and joyful relationships that arise in the context of crisis can thrive as you move through and beyond your illness. When the time is right, shed the role of vulnerable and needy patient, and enjoy rich relationships that revel in the joys of good health.

Who has shown you kindness and caring? How are people reaching out to you? How can you reach out to them when needed?

Finding Purpose

Imagine that you wake up one morning and discover that someone shaved your head while you were sleeping. Upon realizing that you are bald for no good reason, you would probably feel any combination of anger, humiliation, frustration, impotence, and sadness. Now imagine that you are receiving chemotherapy and you wake up one morning and discover that your hair is falling out. You may still feel sad, but you may also feel elements of relief ("The treatments are working on my body"), pride ("I am a survivor!"), strength ("I'm willing to lose my hair to get better"), and gratitude ("I'm thankful they have this treatment to help me"). Linked with a sense of purpose, your baldness becomes more tolerable, which can help you feel happier than you might feel otherwise.

A sense of purpose can reshape your survivorship in joyful ways. Knowing the reason behind your procedures and treatments can help you get through them. And, knowing your role—your purpose—in the procedure helps. Each time I undergo scans to follow the status of my lymphoma, my job is to hold still and help the technician take good-quality pictures. If I fulfill my purpose, I'll only have to go through one set of scans and my doctors will get the most accurate information.

Purpose can help you through the emotional challenges, too, and thus help you recapture joy. If you see the purpose behind sharing your negative emotions, you may find the courage to do so. Facing your fears can weaken them and give you courage, as discussed in chapter 7. Seeing the value—the purpose—behind asking for and accepting assistance may help you overcome your reluctance to expose your vulnerabilities or lean on others.

During the years when my cancer kept recurring and I struggled with fear and grief, part of me wanted to stick my head in the sand and not talk about any of it. But I felt a powerful sense of purpose—namely, to love, support, and teach my children—and I knew that I'd do a better job of raising my kids if I received some professional help dealing with my emotions. I hated going to counseling and resented using an hour when my time felt threatened. Already in pain, I was reluctant to bring up emotionally charged topics. Yet, my sense of purpose gave me the courage to go to the office of the hospital social worker and do the hardest work I've ever done. My emotional growth helped my husband and children, and it freed me to pursue happiness during and after treatment.

Your sense of purpose provides the direction and fortitude needed during treatment and recovery. Chances are you will enjoy a more satisfying sense of control and accomplishment with each little step forward if a sense of purpose motivates you to comply with treatment, eat well, get rest, exercise, ask questions, and keep your health-care team informed of changes and problems. By helping you obtain sound knowledge, find hope, and take proper action, purpose makes your journey easier and safer, and, thus, happier.

What is the purpose behind each of your tests and procedures? What is the purpose—the goal—of your treatment? What is the purpose of your discussions with doctors, nurses, friends, family? What is the purpose of each action you are taking to get better or make things better?

Repairing Yourself; Repairing the World

Thinking about the grander questions of the purpose of life can be healing and may bring you happiness, too. Until my own diagnosis, existential questions about the meaning of life and my purpose on earth were quickly quelled with the pat answer "I'm a physician who helps people." Certainly any god, if there is a god, would be pleased, don't you think? In the weeks following my original diagnosis, existential questions took on great urgency, including "What is the meaning of life? Why are we here?"

While wrestling with my fear of dying young, I had many anxiety-induced and medication-tampered dreams. The varied details always faded within seconds of awakening, but their collective message was unshakable: The purpose of life is to help others. This lesson was complemented by one offered by a deeply spiritual Christian friend who survived a chemo-related crisis. After awakening from her coma, she spent her remaining months on earth sharing what she'd seen on the edge: Our purpose is to let God's goodness flow through us.

Maybe these insights and inspiration came directly from God. Maybe they were simply the soulless expression of the complex neurochemical workings of a drugged and stressed brain. Whatever they were, for me the notions of helping others and letting goodness flow through me feel perfectly "right." What cancer taught me—helped me know with my heart as well as my intellect—is that my life is barely a blink in time. I have no doubt that one hundred years from now, let alone a thousand years from now, not a single person will remember my laugh and not a single phrase of mine will remain in print. The only remembrance of me will be a faint echo, a totally unidentifiable ripple effect from my words and actions. This perception of my own insignificance has had the paradoxical effect of energizing me with the power of participating in "Tikun Olam," the Jewish call to repair the world. If you and I, in our short lifetimes, highlight our similarities and not our differences, and if we "love thy neighbor as thyself," our words and actions can be like water droplets dripping over granite. Imperceptibly through the generations, we can help reshape the world into one of love and peace. Before my illness, I watched the news reports and saw a world broken in so many places. It seemed overwhelming. Hopeless. Then I experienced the kindness and caring of hundreds of people who helped me through my illness, and I knew: There is hope, one drop at a time. Hope lies in each of us pursuing our purpose in *all* the worlds we touch—family, community, country, and universe.

Facing my mortality challenged my long-held beliefs about my personal purpose on earth. As a teen, I heard my calling to be a healer and appreciated the power of purpose to clear a straight path through all the confusing and tempting choices and confer a sense of control. Over the years that followed, my commitment to medicine energized me, and my work as a physician brought many rewards. What I didn't realize was that mine was unreflected purpose, and glaringly incomplete. It was only in my undeniable smallness, aloneness, and lack of control as a cancer patient that my eyes were opened to faint possibilities, and my heart to faith. I now believe that medicine is but a sliver of my purpose. If I live with purpose—if all my words are said with purpose, and all my actions are done with purpose—I open the opportunity to participate in the repair of the world. Purpose lies in every word and action, for it is not just *what* we do that helps repair the world but also *how* we do what we do. At times, my purpose may be just to be.

> At times, your purpose may be just to be.

I can't imagine living without purpose. It would be like hugging air. When times are good, purpose keeps me focused, motivated, energized, efficient, and grateful. Purpose makes the joyful times sweeter. And in the tough times, when my dreams are destroyed or my world seems to fall apart, purpose helps me find the strength needed to move forward with hope. Armed with purpose, my disappointments and failures become learning experiences that help me grow stronger. My losses become opportunities to change direction.

A sense of purpose can help you through the challenges of your illness and bring joy into your life even during difficult times. Use your illness as an opportunity to think about your purpose and find meaning in your life.

What are you discovering about your purpose?

Conclusion

Life is good even when it is not what you expect or want or hope for. Life is good even when life is hard. You can't always choose your circumstances, but you can always choose how you deal with them. By definition, once you are handed a diagnosis, you are a survivor. What kind of survivor do you want to be?

The week after my diagnosis of cancer, I learned that the Chinese word for crisis is composed of two characters: one for danger and one for opportunity. Instinctively, I believed that my illness could be an opportunity. At the very least, experiencing life $\quad$ Life is good. on the other side of the stethoscope would teach me how to become a better doctor. I trusted I'd find more. I hoped there was more. As my survivorship unfolded over the next fourteen years, there *was* more.

If you arc just starting out on your survivorship journey, let me emphasize that the so-called opportunities of my illness have not been welcoming. For a long time, I denied or fought much of my fear, grief, and pain. Strands of pessimism and unhappiness shaded my outlook. Aiming for a certain set of beliefs is one thing; living that belief system is a different matter altogether. I believed my trademark inscription, "There is always hope," during times when my own hope waned like a fickle friend. Even knowing that I'd have to accept uncertainty as a necessary step on my path to happiness, I had difficulty quieting my own anxiety over my not-knowing. It took me ages more than I like to admit before I could let go of my desire to feel in control of the outcome of my illness.

For me, as for most people, Healthy Survivorship and finding happiness are hard work. First you have to put in the time and effort to learn about the skills needed, and then you have to practice and practice until your skills become second nature. Survivorship offers innumerable opportunities to develop and test your ability to be a Healthy Survivor and find happiness.

Healing comes easier to some than to others. I had to travel miles for trials and slog through stressful times at home. And, yes, it was worth every drop of blood, sweat, and tears. By the mid 1990s, although I was still dealing with cancer, I was enjoying a state of hopeful acceptance. I expected to need more cancer treatment every year or so for the rest of my life, while I continued hoping and praying for a lasting remission. Controlling all I could and letting go of all I couldn't led me to a sense of peacefulness and wholeness that made my life happier no matter what was happening medically. Except for rare moments of crisis, my life has never been totally defined by cancer; illness has been just one part of my life, a life that has included joy.

Now my scans are normal. Cheers! It's been over six years since my last treatment. Although my extraordinary recovery remains somewhat of a mystery today, I expect researchers one day hence will have the technology and information to look back at my medical history and explain in scientific terms exactly why my particular cancer gradually disappeared after my eighth course of treatment and never came back. And they will use this knowledge to cure patients newly diagnosed with similar cancers.

For eight years, I was a cancer patient who needed definitive answers about my disease before medical science was ready with any. So I did the next best thing: I obtained sound knowledge about healing after cancer; I received the best treatments that science had to offer; I nourished hope while tending to all my various medical and nonmedical needs; and I lived my life as well as I could. Sometimes it meant getting sicker in order to get better. Sometimes it meant crying in order to laugh, and leaning on others in order to become independent. Healthy Survivorship demanded that I explore unpleasant territory so that I could learn how to move beyond it. On the good days and the rough ones, and after uplifting successes and discouraging disappointments, I did the best I could.

During those years, while researchers were unraveling the mysteries and looking for better answers for patients with my type of lymphoma, I got well. Recoveries happen even when we aren't exactly sure why. If medicine hasn't yet found sure cures for what ails you, don't despair. You can stack the odds in your favor by obtaining sound knowledge, finding and nourishing hope, and taking effective action. You can heal.

What about your happiness? You are the captain of your boat, charting the course of your life in challenging seas. At the helm of a ship far from shore, is it possible to feel happy or be happy when an unpredicted hurricane blows with gale force? Can you feel happy when your ship is being tossed about by dangerously high swells? Probably not, if you aren't wearing foul-weather gear or you don't even know that such protection exists. Surely not, if you have no idea how to adjust the sails and rudders when the wind changes or waves are crashing onboard, or if you don't trust your crew to respond. Your fear and confusion would lead to helplessness and hopelessness that amplify every crack of thunder and rise of the boat's bow. Instinct might drive you to respond in ways that don't help your situation, and might even make things worse. "I'm going to die" may be the only conscious thought that breaks through.

It doesn't have to be this way. With knowledge of your boat and the ways of the sea, you can stay focused and confident, respecting both the forces against you and your ability to ride out the storm. Protected from the elements by state-of-the-art coverings and empowered by expertise and experience, your encounter with nature becomes a game of wits and endurance as you respond appropriately to every shift in the wind and every rogue wave and to whatever other problems occur along the way.

Treatment and recovery can be harsh. When you are going through diagnostic tests, taking rigorous treatments, or dealing with side effects or aftereffects, you may feel traumatized. Being a patient in a complex and high-tech medical system can make you feel powerless. You are not. Think of a captain who, instead of feeling victimized by rough seas, feels *determined* and *empowered*. Confidently busy, he focuses on the tasks at hand such as battening down the hatches, pumping water from the flooded deck, or repairing a piece of equipment that has torn loose. If the best course of action is to steer directly into the waves, the captain orders his crew to ride the bucking storm, encouraging them: "Let's go!" Life is not a problem to be avoided but an adventure to be embraced. You can feel determined and empowered, too, by taking charge of your journey.

You can't be happy all the time. Even experienced veterans find it impossible to feel happy while watching a forty-foot wave threaten to capsize their boat. But during a storm a captain might feel gloriously at one with his crew as they all carry out their tasks, and he might stop and look with awe as lightning streaks brilliantly across the sky. Happiness can arise out of the electrifying awareness, "I am alive!" while you are engaged in extraordinary efforts to survive the forces of nature. From the time of your diagnosis on, you can marvel at the miracles of modern medicine and technology that are helping your body heal. Savor the love flowing to and from the people supporting your journey. And in the relative calm of waiting for treatments to work and for your pain and disease to relent, take comfort in the knowledge that your storm will pass.

No storm lasts forever. Sound knowledge and genuine hope can help you guide your ship through the storm, and love of life can lead you to happiness. After the rain stops and the winds die down, may you ease into safe harbor and use the lessons learned to enrich your life today, tomorrow, and every single day.

Hope

Hope is *an image of goals*
planted firmly in your mind.
When looking at life before you,
hope lines the paths you find.

Hope is *a well of courage*
nestled deep within your heart.
When faltering in fear and doubt,
hope pushes you to start.

Hope is *an urge to keep going,*
for limbs too tired and weak.
When apathy stills all desire,
hope sparks the fuel you seek.

Hope is *a promise of patience*
as you wait for distress to wane.
When all you can do is nothing,
hope pulls you through the pain.

Hope is *a spirit that lifts you,*
should heaviness pull at your soul.
When torn apart by losses,
hope mends to keep you whole.

Appendix I:
Variations on a Theme
by Niebuhr

The opening verse of the ever-popular "Serenity Prayer," which some people call the "Courage Prayer," brought me comfort and inspiration during the months of my initial treatments. Over the years, as I've tried to become a Healthy Survivor, I've taken the liberty of adding verses to help me face the challenges of treatment and long-term survivorship. With credit to Niebuhr's work and a Talmudic proverb, here is a prayer that helps me heal.

God, grant me the . . .

serenity to accept the things I cannot change,
courage to change the things I can,
and wisdom to know the difference.

patience to wait when healing requires time,
courage to undergo more treatment when needed,
and wisdom to know the difference.

discipline to weigh good options,
courage to reject bad advice,
and wisdom to know the difference.

freedom to nourish realistic hopes,
courage to abandon false hopes,
and wisdom to know the difference.

composure to trust my doctors and nurses when they have all they need,
courage to question my doctors and nurses when they may need more,
and wisdom to know the difference.

determination to be independent when I can,
courage to ask for help when required,
and wisdom to know the difference.

power to repress upsetting thoughts that only hurt,
courage to work through upsetting thoughts that can help,
and wisdom to know the difference.

stamina to keep pushing when it can improve the outcome,
courage to adjust when now is the best it can be,
and wisdom to know the difference.

energy to be with people who care,
courage to avoid people who pull me down,
and wisdom to know the difference.

persistence to pursue goals that inspire,
courage to let go of dreams that only frustrate,
and wisdom to know the difference.

flexibility to shift direction from a failing approach,
courage to stay the course when it deserves more time,
and wisdom to know the difference.

vision to appreciate what remains,
courage to grieve what's been lost,
and wisdom to know the difference.

humility to pray as if everything depends on you,
courage to act as if everything depends on me,
and wisdom to do both.

Appendix II:
Language of Healthy Survivorship

How you talk about yourself and your survivorship affects how you feel about yourself and your life. The language of Healthy Survivorship uses words and ideas that help you get good care and live fully. It fosters self-confidence, comfort, perseverance, courage, and hope. Find words and phrases that help you think about your survivorship in life-enhancing ways.

1. Use phrases that acknowledge your challenges while leaving room for hope.

When you feel like saying:	**Try saying:**
"My treatment is *too* hard."	"My treatment is *very* hard."
"This is *too* stressful"	"This is *very* stressful."
"I am *too* afraid."	"I am *very* afraid."
"I'll *never* feel whole again."	"I don't feel whole *right now*."
"It is *impossible*."	"I *need help* finding a solution."
"I *can't* take any more."	"I *need* help to deal with this."

2. Use phrases that reframe your losses in positive ways.

When you feel like saying:	Try saying:
"The treatment is worse than the disease."	"This rough treatment is better than my disease being out of control."
"This treatment gives me *only* a fifty-fifty chance of a good outcome."	"This treatment increases my chances a lot for a good outcome."
"The surgeons are carving me up."	"The surgeons are repairing my problem."
"My medical problems are running my life."	"Managing my medical problems is a full-time job right now."

3. Use phrases that correct myth and misinformation.

When people say:	Remember:
"Your disease is incurable."	There are no incurable diseases; only diseases for which scientists are working toward cures. If your disease has no known cures, remember that it is still treatable.
"You failed your treatment."	You didn't fail your treatment; your treatment failed you.
"It is hopeless."	There is always hope, and you have a right to be hopeful.

Appendix III:
Tips for Being an Effective Patient

You get better care when you help your physicians and nurses care for you, so here are some tips to help you be an effective patient.

- Come prepared for your doctor visits. Call ahead if you are not sure if you are supposed to be fasting, to be bringing something, or to be taking or refraining from certain medications. Bring a list of every medication you are taking, prescription and nonprescription. Bring your list of questions and concerns.
- Be honest about your symptoms or problems. Reporting symptoms is not complaining. Wanting an understandable explanation of your illness or treatment is not "wasting" anyone's time.
- Trust your doctor. If you don't, find a doctor whom you do trust.
- Learn when you need to call the doctor's office and when a noticeable change or a problem can wait. If you are unsure about calling (even if it's 2 A.M.), call and let the doctor or nurse decide if it needs attention. Better to be safe than sorry.
- Keep your physicians aware of your concerns regarding your physical, psychological, emotional, or spiritual situations.
- Inform your physicians if there is a problem with a physician or staff member. Give specific examples.

- Make it clear to your physicians the limits, if any, of how much information you want shared with your family.
- Leave the doctor's office only *after* you are clear about all your instructions, prescriptions, appointments, tests, treatments, or follow-up calls. Do not depend on the office or hospital to call and remind you.
- If you think you are supposed to be scheduled for a test and the office has not scheduled it or seems to know nothing about it, ask the staff to check with your doctor. Do not assume that the test was canceled or that you were in error.
- Make sure you get all your test results (blood work, scans, biopsies, etc.). Do NOT assume that no news is good news.
- If your doctors are running late because they are with other patients, remind yourself that your doctors are spending time with patients who need them. One day, that patient might be you, and you'll be glad that your doctor takes the time needed to tend to you.

Appendix IV:
Tips for Preventing Medication Problems

The following tips supplement those presented on pages 171–72 of chapter 6 for preventing problems related to your medications.

1. Find out more about the known risks associated with the drug.

- Talk with your doctors, nurses, and pharmacist.
- Ask your doctor or pharmacist for a patient information sheet.
- Visit a reputable Web site.
  - www.fda.gov has links to a tab for "drug information" that provides a link to a section on "drug safety and side effects."
  - www.drugdigest.org is a free Web site that allows you to check for drug interactions with any of the drugs you are already taking.
  - www.pubmed.gov contains abstracts citations from professional journals.
- Read the entry for the drug in the *PDR, Physician's Desk Reference.*

2. Review with your physician(s) any possible increased risk of the medication *for you* related to

- all your current medical conditions, no matter how minor;

- your current medications (prescription and nonprescription; pills, liquids, suppositories, creams, and patches);
- your past medical history (e.g., past medical conditions, past surgeries, past problems with medications);
- your family history (e.g., medical conditions in family members that might put you at increased risk of developing the same condition);
- your lifestyle (e.g., smoking, alcohol use, illicit drug use, low/high level of physical activity, living alone, and unusual diet);
- special health- or health-care-related needs that might affect the decision about the use of a particular drug (e.g., desire to preserve your fertility or living too far for the frequent blood tests).

Talking with your health-care team about medications is not a social situation. You may be putting yourself at increased risk of side effects and complications if you lie about your smoking, alcohol use, diet, contraceptives, or use of alternative therapies. I cannot emphasize enough how important it is to *make sure* your doctors are aware of every single prescription and nonprescription drug you take, no matter how infrequently you take it, and any other factors that might affect the safety of a new drug.

An ounce of prevention is worth a pound of cure.

Appendix V:
The Patient's Bill of Rights

The Patient's Bill of Rights was first adopted by the American Hospital Association (AHA) in 1973 and revised in October 1992. The AHA encourages hospitals, health-care institutions, and all health-care workers to use these as a guideline. Patients can exercise these rights on their own behalf or by a designated substitute decision-maker if a patient can no longer make decisions for himself or herself or if the patient is a minor.

Patient's Rights

- You have the right to considerate and respectful care.
- You have the right to obtain from the members of your health-care team information about your diagnosis, treatment, and prognosis that is relevant, current, and understandable.
- Except in emergencies when you lack the ability to make decisions and your need for treatment is urgent, you are entitled to an opportunity to discuss and request information related to the specific procedures and/or treatments available, the risks involved, the possible length of recovery, and the medically reasonable alternatives to existing treatments along with their accompanying risks and benefits.
- You have the right to know the identity of all physicians, nurses, and

others involved in your care, as well as when those involved are students, residents, or other trainees. You also have the right to know the immediate and long-term financial significance of treatment choices insofar as they are known.

- You have the right to make decisions about the plan of care before and during the course of treatment and to refuse a recommended treatment or plan of care if it is permitted by law and hospital policy. You have the right to be informed of the medical consequences of this action. In case of such refusal, you are still entitled to appropriate care and services that the hospital provides or to be transferred to another hospital. The hospital should notify you of any policy at the other hospital that might affect your choice.

- You have the right to have an advance directive (such as a living will, health-care proxy, or durable power of attorney for health care) concerning treatment or designating a surrogate decision-maker and to expect that the hospital will honor that directive as permitted by law and hospital policy.

- Health-care institutions must advise you of your rights under state law and hospital policy to make informed medical choices, must ask if you have an advance directive, and must include that information in your medical records. You have the right to know about any hospital policy that may keep it from carrying out a legally valid advance directive.

- You have the right to privacy. Case discussion, consultation, examination, and treatment should be conducted to protect your privacy.

- You have the right to expect that all communications and records pertaining to your care will be treated confidentially by the hospital, except in cases such as suspected abuse and public-health hazards when reporting is permitted or required by law. You have the right to expect that the hospital will emphasize confidentiality of this information when it releases it to any other parties entitled to review information in these records.

- You have the right to review your medical records and to have the information explained or interpreted as necessary, except when restricted by law.

- You have the right to expect that, within its capacity and policies, a hospital will make reasonable response to your request for appropriate and medically indicated care and services. The hospital must provide evaluation, service, and/or referral as indicated by the urgency of the case. When medically appropriate and legally permissible, or when you have so requested, you may be transferred to another facility. The institution to which you are to be transferred must first have accepted you for transfer. You also must have the benefit of complete information and explanation concerning the need for, risks, benefits, and alternatives to such a transfer.

- You have the right to ask and be told of the existence of any business relationship among the hospital, educational institutions, other health-care providers, and/or payers that may influence your treatment and care.
- You have the right to consent to or decline to participate in proposed research studies or human experimentation and to have those studies fully explained before you consent. If you decline to participate in research or experimentation, you are still entitled to the most effective care that the hospital can otherwise provide.
- You have the right to expect reasonable continuity of care and to be informed by physicians and other caregivers of available and realistic patient-care options when hospital care is no longer appropriate.
- You have the right to be informed of hospital policies and practices that relate to patient care, treatment, and responsibilities. You have the right to be informed of available resources for resolving disputes, grievances, and conflicts, such as ethics committees, patient representatives, or other mechanisms available in the institution. You have the right to be informed of the hospital's charges for services and available payment methods.

The effectiveness of your care and your satisfaction with the course of treatment depends, in part, on you fulfilling certain responsibilities.

Patient's Responsibilities

- You are responsible for providing information about past illnesses, hospitalizations, medications, and other health-related matters.
- You must take responsibility for requesting additional information or

clarification about your health status or treatment when you do not fully understand the current information or instructions.

- You are responsible for making sure that the health-care institution has a copy of your written advance directive if you have one.
- You are responsible for informing your physicians and other caregivers if you anticipate problems in following prescribed treatment.
- You also should be aware that the hospital has to be reasonably efficient and equitable in providing care to other patients and the community. The hospital's rules and regulations are designed to help the hospital meet this obligation.
- You and your family are responsible for being considerate of and making reasonable accommodations to the needs of the hospital, other patients, medical staff, and hospital employees.
- You are responsible for providing necessary information for insurance claims and for working with the hospital as needed to make payment arrangements.
- You are responsible for recognizing the impact of your lifestyle on your personal health.

Appendix VI:
Support Groups

Recent research has shown that many people's level of stress, ability to cope, and quality of life improve with participation in a well-designed and supervised support group. In general, groups led by a qualified health professional offer certain advantages, such as keeping the group discussion on track, preventing disruptions, and recognizing participants who need one-on-one therapy. Regarding support groups for children, it is even more important to make sure the group is facilitated by a qualified health-care professional. If a particular type of support is not helping, you can stop at any time.

The advantages of attending a support group include
- providing a place where your illness is "normal" and the focus is on living well;
- providing a place to laugh and find joy in hard times;
- preventing or diminishing your sense of isolation;
- providing a safe place to discuss your thoughts and feelings;
- easing the burden on family and friends, especially if your illness is chronic;
- enabling you to keep some issues private from family and friends;
- opening opportunities to learn helpful tips about treatment options;

- exposure to a variety of effective coping styles for getting through treatment, dealing with co-workers or family, and other aspects of living with illness;
- motivating you to take effective action;
- helping you to find meaning in hard times;
- providing an opportunity to "give back," even while dealing with illness;
- bolstering your hope by introducing you to people who have recovered from or have adapted well to similar challenges, recovered despite slim odds, learned to live well with the uncertainty, and found great happiness in their lives.

A support group is helping you if
- you feel comfortable during the meetings;
- you leave the meeting feeling inspired, stronger, understood, less anxious, less lonely, more confident, or more hopeful. (Note: these positive feelings may first arise hours or days *after* the support group meeting.)

A support group may not be a wise choice now if
- you are feeling completely overwhelmed by your illness;
- you can't handle hearing about anyone else's situation or problems right now;
- you feel like hurting yourself or ending it all.

In these cases, call your physicians and *make sure they know how you are feeling,* just as you would call them if you were bleeding or had a high fever. Appropriate attention can help you get through your distress, adjust, and move forward with hope.

To find a support group that meets your needs, choose from groups that
- are open-ended (you go for as many weeks, months, or years as you like);
- closed (you go for a defined number of sessions);
- revolve around one particular disease or medical problem (such as multiple sclerosis, metastatic breast cancer, colostomy);
- revolve around one type of treatment (such as bone marrow transplant);
- revolve around one social situation (such as under age 40, particular religious affiliation).

Find out about available support groups by calling
- your doctor's office;
- your hospital's social service department;
- the local chapter of national disease-specific organizations;
- local wellness organizations such as Gilda's Club or Wellness Community.

Online Support Groups

A variety of online and telephone support services are now available. Besides being free of charge, advantages include
- access 24 hours a day, 7 days a week;
- ability to participate in the privacy of your home;
- the opportunity to listen anonymously (without ever having to contribute to discussion);
- access to an almost unlimited variety of people and situations—higher likelihood of finding someone very similar to yourself;
- wide assortment of online presentations: chat rooms, discussion boards, collections of personal stories and discussions, prerecorded presentations and interviews.

Avoid the dangers of online support groups by
- never giving your personal information (such as phone, address, social security numbers);
- never ordering therapies recommended by an online group;
- staying connected with your friends and family at home (don't shut them out after you find companionship and understanding from your online friends);
- always discussing with your doctor any information that conflicts with what you've been told or when a different therapy is recommended.

Never pursue ANY medical treatment recommended in any in-person or online support setting without discussing fully with your physicians first.

Index